May 2016

MOBILE SERVICES

THE TRUTH ABOUT EXERCISE ADDICTION

THE TRUTH ABOUT EXERCISE ADDICTION

Understanding the Dark Side of Thinspiration

Katherine Schreiber and Heather A. Hausenblas

ROWMAN & LITTLEFIELD
Lanham • Boulder • New York • London

Published by Rowman & Littlefield
A wholly owned subsidary of The Rowman & Littlefield Publishing Group,
Inc.
4501 Forbes Boulevard, Suite 200, Lanham, Maryland 20706
www.rowman.com

Unit A, Whitacre Mews, 26–34 Stannary Street, London SE11 4AB, United
Kingdom

British Library Cataloguing in Publication Information Available

Library of Congress Cataloging-in-Publication Data

Schreiber, Katherine, 1988–
The truth about exercise addiction : understanding the dark side of thinspiration / Katherine
Schreiber and Heather A. Hausenblas.
pages cm
Includes bibliographical references and index.
ISBN 978-1-4422-3329-4 (cloth : alk. paper)—ISBN 978-1-4422-3330-0 (electronic)
1. Exercise addiction. 2. Eating disorders. I. Hausenblas, Heather A. II. Title.
RC569.5.E94S37 2015
613.7'1—dc23
2014030124

∞™ The paper used in this publication meets the minimum requirements of
American National Standard for Information Sciences Permanence of Paper
for Printed Library Materials, ANSI/NISO Z39.48-1992.

Printed in the United States of America

CONTENTS

ACKNOWLEDGMENTS

Katherine thanks Sandy Marks for his love, support, and impeccable patience—all of which has inspired her to maintain hope and inspiration throughout the writing of this book.

She also thanks David Tao, Zachary Sniderman, and Derek Flanzraich for letting the seeds of this book take root on Greatist.com. This book would not have been possible without the enthusiastic, insightful, and immensely helpful input from Jodi Rubin, Angie Lockwood, Carolyn Costin, Lara Pence, Judith Brisman, and Keri Peterson.

Infinite thanks to Kaila Prins, Charlotte Andersen, Colleen Siti, Myles Alexander, Ben Carter, Arielle Norman, Marion Maclean, Jennifer Hicks, Emily Duncan, Kate Hanisko, "B," and Catherine Goldberg for their bravery and openness in sharing their experiences. May you all succeed in your recovery efforts and know that your stories will inspire many others.

Most importantly, Katherine thanks Heather Hausenblas for her enthusiasm, willingness, and collaboration on this needed resource. Much gratitude is also due to Suzanne Staszak-Silva, our editor, whose interest and careful eye enabled this book to come into being. Many, many thanks to Stephanie Sculetti for moving this book forward, step by step. And a standing ovation to Erin McGarvey for her phenomenal copyediting job and unparalleled attention to detail.

Heather thanks the many undergraduate and graduate students and colleagues who have inspired her and taught her so much about the psychology of health during the last twenty years. In particular, Danielle Symons Downs, her former graduate student and now treasured colleague, with whom she spent countless hours developing the Exercise Dependence Scale, entering data, and trying to understand how people can become addicted to exercise.

A special thank you to our editor Suzanne Staszak-Silva. Her support and insight made this book possible.

Heather also thanks her husband, Todd, and three boys, Tommy, Scotty, and Johnny, for making every day an adventure filled with love.

Finally, Heather extends her highest gratitude to Katherine Schreiber, who reached out in June 2013 to provide insight into an article she was writing on exercise addiction. Heather instantly liked her contagious enthusiasm for trying to understand exercise addiction. Two months later Heather and Katherine began to write this book together. Katherine was the main driving force in getting this book completed—her unstoppable work ethic and passion are an inspiration.

Heather dedicates this book to Bert Carron, an incredible mentor and friend. His spirit, vitality, and passion for his profession will remain in Heather's memory infinitely.

I

WHAT IT IS

Defining Exercise Addiction

Maybe you've noticed a particularly avid exerciser at your fitness club—someone who predictably occupies a cardiovascular machine for noticeably long lengths of time or hovers around the weight room well after others have toweled off and called it a day. Perhaps you've even felt lazy by comparison or in awe of this person's apparent stamina. But did you ever wonder whether his or her ostensibly healthy drive to stay "fit" might be bordering on pathology?

Can people really become addicted to exercise? The answer is yes. But the questions are who, why, how, where, and when.

Exercise addiction is thought to afflict an estimated 3 percent of regular gym-goers.[1, 2, 3] Some research suggests 25 percent of runners qualify as "addicted" to their sport of choice.[4] Among triathletes the prevalence of exercise addiction has been found to top 52 percent.[5] Exercise addiction comes in a variety of shapes and sizes—ranging from bone-thin to explosively buff individuals—and, though most common among those younger than thirty-five,[6] it can strike at any age.

The largest prevalence study to date was conducted with a national representative sample of 2,710 Hungarian adults aged eighteen to sixty-four years.[7] Of this total sample, 474 people reportedly exercised at least once a week. These active folks were asked to complete questionnaires, like the Exercise Dependence Scale (included in appendix B and discussed in chapter 2, "What It Looks Like: The Signs and Symptoms of Exercise Addiction"), which assessed how addictive their relationship to working out was. Researchers analyzed the physically active participants' reports of time spent in motion, sport of choice, and attitudes surrounding exercise in addition to the lifestyle reports from their sedentary counterparts and concluded that an estimated 0.3 percent of the total population was at risk for exercise addiction. These research-based estimates are in concordance with the argument that exercise addiction is relatively rare, especially when compared to other addictions.[8] Small as this number may seem, however, it still translates to roughly thirty out of every ten thousand people. Given the physical and emotional consequences associated with these high-risk cases (as you'll learn in chapter 5, "What It Does: The Short- and Long-term Health Risks of Exercise Addiction"), that's no insignificant number.

As far as race and socioeconomic status are concerned, not enough research has been done yet to definitively point toward any trends or predictors. But considering that the risk of exercise addiction is higher among more active groups of people, we can assume that the demographic factors predictive of greater exercise behavior in general would also predict higher rates of exercise addiction.

For instance, it has been found that individuals with higher levels of education engage in more physical activity.[9] These individuals thus may be at a greater risk of exercise addiction than those who have completed fewer years of schooling. Higher median income levels also predict greater access to physical activity settings. Being a minority is statistically linked to less access to physical activity settings.[10] So one can assume that being a minority may predict a lower prevalence of exercise addiction. Considering that most exercise addicts' gym memberships comprise a large part of their life, the cost of such memberships should also be factored in. Those at lower ends of the socioeconomic spectrum may not be able to finance an addiction to exercise simply because they cannot afford the membership, equipment, and accoutrements (from running shoes to energy bars to yoga gear, weights, exercise classes— you name it!) that a high commitment to exercise often calls for.

That being said, race and socioeconomic factors are by no means inflexible barriers to developing overzealous passions for exercise (or not). But the likelihood of a full-blown addiction to physical activity cropping up may be weaker among individuals with less education and at lower ends of the socioeconomic spectrum.

Exercise addiction is a pattern of physical activity that exceeds what most fitness and medical professionals consider "normal," causes immense psychological anguish (either during, following, or in anticipation of exercise), engulfs an exercise addict's personal, professional, and social life, and is experienced by the addict as difficult to control or reduce in frequency—even in the face of illness or injury.

It is a self-perpetuating craving for movement that results in uncontrollably excessive physical exertion and manifests in mental and physiological distress.[11] If a person reports feelings of anxiety and depression when unable to exercise, spends little or no time with family or friends because of physical activity involvement, or continues to run despite a doctor's advice to allow an overuse injury to heal, he or she could be considered at high risk for exercise addiction.

Exercise addicts experience physical activity as both a coping mechanism and a compulsion without which they feel they cannot survive. In addition to exercising despite injury and illness, they experience a certain type of withdrawal when they are not able to work out as planned (or if they miss a gym session or jog). The prospect of taking one or more "off days" provokes anxiety in the exercise addict's mind, coupled with guilt, irritability, depression, fatigue, and occasionally even physical aches or pains in the event he or she skips a planned exercise session.

Social, occupational, and family obligations are sidelined in the exercise addict's day-to-day existence, as ad nauseam strength or endurance training takes precedence over all else.[12] More often than not, the pathological levels of exertion that the exercise addict seeks play into, exacerbate, or destructively inspire body image disturbances and/or eating disorders.

Like all potentially addictive substances or behaviors, exercise has the distinctive feature of—in addition to temporarily alleviating psychological distress—flooding our brains with positive feelings.[13] Exercise in overdrive fulfills this criterion, boosting our bodies' natural neurochemical painkillers (beta-endorphins), while simultaneously dialing down anxiety, dispelling anger, quieting our minds, and transiently buoying our self-esteem. Physical activity's ability to grant us this mental and physical release and euphoria is precisely what renders it so addictive to a select segment of individuals prone to compulsive behavior. Although exercise addicts experience less pleasure as a consequence of developing a tolerance for high levels of exertion atop exhaustion from their relentless pursuit of physical activity "fixes" over time, their initial attraction to working out is fueled by its promise to make them *feel better*. In the long run, "feeling better" becomes less about chasing after that so-called runner's high and more about avoiding intolerable emotions (i.e., anxiety and rage) that infiltrate the exercise addict's awareness when he or she can't get to the gym.

Addictions go a step beyond compulsions due to their hallmark of *tolerance*—that is, needing more of a substance or behavior to achieve its initially desired effects. The obsessive pursuit of control or moral superiority, an unmatched sense of self-acceptance, the promise of weight loss via burned calories, or an escape from mental or physical pain may drive the overzealous exerciser to tirelessly seek his or her activity of choice. As long as the amount of time spent performing this behavior remains in check, the exhaustive engagement in exercise can still be couched as compulsion alone. But when the time and frequency of the behavior must be increased in order to achieve whatever mental and physical ease it initially brought about, addiction can be said to have taken hold. Put simply: if an exerciser requires lengthier and/or more frequent bouts of movement to feel that sense of "being okay" in his or her skin, that's a red flag for addiction, elevating what may have begun as a compulsive behavior to a higher severity. For the exercise addict, this means the initial thirty-minute cardio session that used to calm him or her down no longer suffices. A minimum of forty-five minutes may become necessary, progressing over time to an hour or more before she or he can feel calm enough to attend to non-exercise-related obligations.

Another difference between compulsions and addictions entails how realistic the feared consequences of not performing a coveted behavior (or procuring a preferred substance) are. Concerns that arise when a compulsive behavior cannot be performed tend to be less realistic than the feared consequences associated with not engaging in addictive behaviors. For example, an individual who feels the compulsion to check his stove's gas light six times prior to leaving his apartment may have an irrational fear that his home will burn to ash if he doesn't painstakingly preempt a fire. An exercise addict, by contrast, has a more realistic fear of the negative mood, increased anxiety, fatigue, and deflated sense of accomplishment he knows he'll experience on days his gym routines are stymied. In other words: the exercise addict fears the very real feeling of withdrawal if he or she can't get that physical activity "fix." Even if deemed objectively trivial or outlandish by those who cannot grasp the interiority of the exercise addict's mind, the apprehension exercise addicts feel in anticipation of not being able to work out is rooted in a very real physiological and emotional response.

Many exercise addicts also experience overblown fears that they will "get fat" or lose too much muscle tone in the event they cannot work out as planned. These exaggerated phobias of weight gain or weight loss have been linked, not surprisingly, to fundamentally flawed senses of self-esteem, identity disturbances, and impaired abilities to self-soothe.[14] The rate of eating disorders among those who use exercise in a pathological manner is substantial. Nearly half of all individuals diagnosed with an eating disorder are thought to suffer from a dangerously severe number of exercise addiction symptoms.[15] To differentiate between those who abuse exercise to aid and abet an eating disorder (also known as secondary exercise addicts) and those who obsessively work out without a primary concern over weight loss or weight gain (also known as primary exercise addicts), researchers studying pathological pursuits of physical activity often administer measures assessing fears of fat or body dysmorphia (like the Goldfarb Fear of Fat Scale).[16] These tools enable psychologists to determine what's really motivating self-destructive levels of repetitive exertion. Exercise addicts who suffer from accompanying eating disorders tend to experience even greater degrees of psychological turmoil—not to mention physical consequences due to malnutrition, as we'll explore further in chapter 5.

Both rational and irrational fears alike fuel the exercise addict's destructive adherence to physical exertion, as does a deep-seated terror of losing hold on an activity that gradually becomes his or her sole means of deriving empowerment and self-esteem. (See chapter 6, "Why It Happens," for more about the hidden motivations to balk at off days and hurl oneself into endless cycles of sweating.) Compulsion (*I must get to the gym or else*), all-or-nothing thought processes (i.e., *If I don't lift/run/stretch enough, I will lose something that renders me valuable or important* or *If I don't complete my workout routine I won't be able to focus*), social isolation, and high levels of anxiety warp the exercise addict's mind as his or her disorder progresses, reinforcing him- or herself with each compulsively pursued exercise session, feeding off low self-esteem, and perpetuating a narrowed mind-set that simultaneously considers the relentless pursuit of physical activity as both *savior from* and *source of* abject misery.

A NOTE ABOUT LANGUAGE: WHY WE'VE CHOSEN THE "EXERCISE ADDICTION" LABEL

There's debate within the mental health field regarding how to label overzealous pursuits of physical activity. Some argue in favor of calling it "compulsive" exercise, others, "obligatory" or "obsessive" exercise. Labels like *bigorexia* have also been bandied about to describe the relentless pursuit of increased size and strength.

Below is a list of the eighteen most commonly used terms to de-scribe exercise in overdrive—in psych lit and popular media:

- Exercise addiction
- Bodybuilder addiction
- Negative addiction
- Running addiction
- Attitudinal commitment
- Exercise commitment
- Running commitment
- Obsessive commitment
- Exercise dependence
- Excessive exercise
- Fitness fanaticism
- Obligatory exercise
- Compulsive running
- Chronic jogging
- Habitual running
- High-intensity running
- Running dependence

- Obligatory running

Some professionals shy away from labeling the drive to work out beyond normal or recommended levels as an "addiction" for fear of lumping what they consider to be mere "behavioral" compulsions into the same category as substance abuse. Those who avoid the term "addiction" in reference to excessive exercise argue that the criteria for substance addictions are too distinct from compulsivity to warrant comparison. Going cold turkey on your gym sessions might make you angry, frustrated, anxious, and fatigued, for instance, but it won't necessarily induce tremors or hallucinations as ceasing to drink after months of regularly imbibing five or more alcoholic beverages per day would.

Indeed, the only behavior qualifying as addictive in the most recent edition of the American Psychiatric Association's *Diagnostic and Statistical Manual of Mental Disorders*[17] is excessive gambling. Per the American Psychiatric Association, all other potentially addictive behaviors—not just exercise, but sex, Internet browsing, and shopping—require further research before unequivocally standing as uniquely diagnosable pathologies. (So stay tuned!)

When scrutinized closely, however, the criteria currently in place to describe drug and alcohol addiction are strikingly applicable to pathological pursuits of exercise—as we'll see in chapter 2.

Exercise addiction has also been framed as a form of dependence. Functionally, dependence and addiction refer to the same pattern of behavior—namely, the body's physiological adaptation to repeated doses of a substance (or repeated iterations of a behavior) such that the amount of the substance (or frequency of the behavior) must be increased to achieve its initial effects.

Some types of substance use (e.g., prescription drug use, nonproblematic alcohol use) may show tolerance or mild withdrawal symptoms without the compulsive elements of a disorder severe enough to qualify as an addiction. The same might be said about the natural tolerance gym-goers build in response to regular strength or aerobic training— they can handle more weight and longer cardio sessions and may indeed experience fatigue, achiness, or irritability on days that they cannot get to the gym. But only when the need to exercise begins dominating their focus, leading to injuries that they persist in trying to work past without rest and inducing more psychological discomfort than less, do such individuals' relationships with exercise begin to raise red flags.

For the purposes of this book, as well as to legitimize a psychological disorder that is often waved off as impossible or unbelievable (*How could something so good for you ever be so bad? Gee, I wish I was addicted to the gym!*), the authors prefer the term *exercise addiction*. Addiction terminology encompasses all forms of problematic exercise, ranging from compulsive to disturbingly craved to out of control.

The authors do not advocate the application of the term "exercise addiction" to a behavior that fails to meet the criteria listed in chapter 2, but they believe it is important to consider exercise addiction as a real and legitimate pathology in order to lend much-needed weight to an often misunderstood and all too readily dismissed psychological disturbance.

2

WHAT IT LOOKS LIKE

The Signs and Symptoms of Exercise Addiction

The more you exercise, the better, right? Research shows that when we increase our activity levels, our mental and physical health follow suit—up to a certain point, that is. When we stop taking "off days," or work out for longer than our bodies can handle, we impair our strength, our stamina, and our overall well-being. By overexerting ourselves, we also risk throwing off our psychological equilibrium.

Although there's a minimum recommended amount of exercise, science hasn't yet figured out an objective upper limit that applies to everyone. Some research suggests exercise's mental benefits max out at around fourteen hours of physical activity per week.[1] But each of has a unique tipping point beyond which continuing to sweat, lift, burn, or push past pain does more harm than good.

Part of knowing this limit is a function of being in touch with our physical and emotional needs (i.e., *if I'm grumpy after my gym sessions, I may not have eaten enough beforehand or adequately refueled after*). Developing a sense of when we should really stop, stretch, and replenish (or rest) is a trial-and-error process that's not exactly straightforward for most people. For those who exercise compulsively (say, to offset anxiety and depression, buoy self-esteem, or, if an eating disorder's involved, purge excess calories), staying in tune with body and mind is even harder.

Exercise helps dispel negative emotions—anger, depression, anxiety, and even boredom can melt away after a mere ten minutes of getting our move on.[2] And it produces those blissful endorphin rushes commonly dubbed "runner's high." (You can thank the segments of our nervous system that regulate pain, reward, and motivation—our body's endogenous opioid system—for that one.) But this very ability to offer escape *and* produce influxes of mood-boosting brain chemicals is precisely what renders physical activity so hard to quit for those prone to addiction. The social validation that hitting the gym typically offers also helps sow the seeds of a hard-to-quit fixation. (*You worked out six times this week? You ran a 5K without stopping? Wow, you're incredible!* Who doesn't want to hear this kind of praise?)

For the exercise addict, what begins as a salutary coping or health-maintenance mechanism easily blossoms into a rigid ritual whose emotional and bodily benefits the addict does not believe he can live without. She may start assuming that the self-acceptance, post-exercise calm, or focus her workouts afford her cannot be achieved by any means other than the daily set of crunches, early morning run, or twice daily speed walks to which she keeps adding reps, kilometers, or minutes.

Her routine may begin to swallow more of her time. Soon she's canceling plans to stay home and perform aerobic routines to the echo of a workout DVD or a down-pat series of private exercises. Or she's riddled with anxiety the weekend her in-laws are in town and she can't spend that full forty-five minutes on the Stairmaster as planned.

Just to circumvent the dysphoria affiliated with missing a workout, the exercise addict may begin ducking out of non-fitness-related obligations—many of which he may have formerly deemed fun. (*Sorry, guys, can't do happy hour today . . . or tomorrow; actually, scratch that dinner, too. Maybe we can try for next week?*)

Soon exercise loses its liberating quality. It becomes the primary—and sometimes sole—means of escaping distress. The discomfort of psychological withdrawal from not going to the gym builds, eclipsing not only the importance, but also the allure of social activities, family demands, or professional pursuits.

Time spent lifting, sweating, exerting, and burning expands. Whereas a fifty-minute cardio and stretch session used to suffice, now the exercise addict requires two hours or more to exit the gym happy. Any less and he can't focus on the next item on his agenda—be that reading for pleasure after a long day at work, brainstorming in a meeting with the rest of his colleagues, or enjoying a movie or live music performance.

The ever-increasing pursuit of fitness at all costs raises the exercise addict's risk of overuse injury. Sprained or strained ligaments, muscle tears, tendinitis, and iliotibial band syndrome are imminent.[3] At the same time the exercise addict may become even more vulnerable to depression,[4] anxiety,[5] amplified body image disturbances,[6] and even the onset of an eating disorder.[7]

Coworkers, friends, and significant others may take notice and suggest she cut back on her workouts, so as to recover from, say, shin splints, or to give an achy back time to heal. Loved ones may point out to the addict that he used to derive so much more joy from life, inquiring whether all this time spent in motion is doing more harm to his health than good.

But to the exercise addict, giving up his preferred mode of coping seems to be too much of a sacrifice. He might have tried to cut back before, only to have met a wave of emotional unease, irritability, sleep disturbances, and even a decreased interest in intimacy. He may attempt to convince his acquaintances—as well as himself—that he's got his habits under control, arguing all the while that exercise is healthy, after all, so how could there be a cause for concern?

Those who find themselves drawn toward pathological levels of physical activity also tend to be actively unaware of (read: averse to acknowledging or seeking the fulfillment of) fundamental bodily and psychological requirements. Sleep, nutrition, social stimuli, and receptivity to care or love along with relaxation and pleasure often strike exercise addicts as threats to their ascetic pursuit of relentless exercise. Describing overzealous athletes in her book *Compulsive Exercise and the Eating Disorders*, psychiatrist Alayne Yates highlights exercise addicts' abject terror "that if they stop . . . running they will collapse, lose their resolve, and fold altogether. What they are saying is that they must hold fast against their very basic human needs."[8]

Exercise addiction doesn't come in just one size. Some individuals may display a tendency to compulsively seek increased strength and muscle while others rigidly adhere to the pursuit of smallness, or weight loss. For many, the mere warding off of anxiety, depression, or other unbearable emotional states undergirds the disorder's characteristically unquenchable urges to remain in motion. The degree and intensity of these cravings or intrusive thoughts often vary among sufferers, with each person falling on a spectrum between at risk and full-blown dependence.

To determine the extent of exercise addicts' suffering, psychologists Heather Hausenblas and Danielle Symons Downs mapped out an assessment tool based on the *Diagnostic and Statistical Manual of Mental Disorders'* criteria for substance dependence. Outlined below, at least three of the following measures must apply to an exerciser for him or her to qualify as addicted.

Those at less disruptive ends of the exercise addiction spectrum identify with three of the symptoms, while those more entrenched in pathology check out on four, five, six, or possibly all:

1. *Tolerance.* The exerciser needs to increase the time spent or the intensity of her preferred mode of physical activity to achieve its originally desired effect (i.e., mood stabilization, enhanced self-esteem, peace of mind, or ability to focus or relax). The amount of exercise that once sufficed no longer makes as much of a difference.

2. *Withdrawal.* In the event a gym-goer can't squeeze in his preferred routine as planned, anxiety skyrockets while anger and frustration often creep in, among other negative emotions, including depression. Fatigue also takes hold, dragging a sufferer's mind-set down further. Addicts may feel compelled to exercise just to offset these unpleasant feelings.

3. *Intention effects.* A hallmark sign of exercise addiction is the repeated intention to work out only for a restricted amount of time, only to find herself exceeding that limit over and over again. Despite planning to spend only thirty minutes on the elliptical or treadmill, an overly enthusiastic exerciser might spend upward of an hour or more in motion, missing or arriving late to an important meeting or event. A weight lifter who promises to stop after three sets (since his stomach's already growling) suddenly feels he can't rest until he's completed a fourth, a fifth, or a sixth. His mind screams at him to push harder, go longer, and avoid stop-

ping—irrespective of his plan to cut himself off at a previously planned-upon limit.

4. *Loss of control.* The worse an exercise addict's pathology becomes, the less of a handle he has over his thoughts, behavior, and response to the gym. Focus outside the gym continually circles back to exercise. Thoughts race to when and how he'll squeeze in his daily routine. Even with an awareness that his regimen may be getting a bit out of hand, the exercise addict repeatedly finds himself unable to stop or cut back. More reps are added and more calories clamor to be burned, even if he wants nothing more than to go home, take a day off, or do something sedentary. Rather than being in control of his workouts, his exercise schedule has assumed control over him.

5. *Time.* A noticeably large chunk of an exercise addict's life is devoted to physical activity. Vacations often revolve around fitness, and downtime may be avoided at all costs. Huge swaths of the exercise addict's days and weeks are allocated to the planning of, engagement in, and recovery from exercise activities. Even when not in motion, the exercise addict may find her attention drifting to thoughts of the gym, concerns about whether she has done enough for the day, or how much longer she has to stay at work before she can escape into the freedom of running, biking, or clicking her shoes into a spin bike come 5:00 pm.

6. *Conflict.* Non-fitness-related activities and roles fall by the wayside—time spent relaxing with friends or quality moments with family are truncated to make more room for exercise. What once brought an exercise addict joy may seem like a nuisance, inasmuch as it gets in the way of his gym routine. Work or academic performance may suffer as a consequence and even more anxiety may accrue in the exercise addict's mind as he becomes torn between fulfilling expectations associated with non-exercise-related obligations and keeping his own ever-increasing cravings for exercise sated.

7. *Continuance.* A strong indicator of exercise addiction is whether a runner, biker, swimmer, yogi, or weight lifter persists in performing her preferred routine despite incurring an injury due to abusing that activity. Continuing to exercise against doctor's orders, in the face of illness, or in spite of aches, pains, fractures, or breaks

indicates pathology. The exerciser has become so disconnected from attending to her body's needs that her motivational system can veritably be considered "hijacked" by an addiction to working out.

Of course, it's not always easy to pinpoint where compulsion splits off from healthy enthusiasm. Most gym-goers, for instance, meet the first criterion—tolerance—since the body naturally adapts to physical activity patterns over time. Whereas ten minutes of jogging used to knock them out at the start of their New Year's resolution, by summertime they can last a full twenty-five minutes.

Even hitting the gym every day or exercising at intensities that makes others say "wow" may not be signs of pathology in and of themselves. Consider the average schedule of a triathlete, who may wake up around 5:00 am to swim three miles before logging an hour-long run before breakfast only to get back on an exercise bike later that afternoon between two carb- and protein-packed meals.

For this person the goal isn't to stave off some gnawing anxiety, to sate an increasing urge to get bigger, or to compensate for eating too much. Nor is a triathlete's schedule designed without the important consideration of adequate rest and recovery days. Rather, the average competitor-in-training adheres to such a rigorous schedule in the interest of reaching his career aspiration—amping up cardiovascular and muscular stamina prior to the next competition under the auspices of trainers, coaches, and, in some cases, nutritional advisers.

In considering triathletes, however, it is important to note that the rates of exercise addiction among these (and other) cohorts of elite-level athletes are far higher than in the average population. One study[9] carried out by Deakin University sports researcher Justin McNamara suggests that as many as 34 percent of top sports competitors display noteworthy exercise addiction symptoms. Another study, conducted by University of Hong Kong sports psychologists Michelle Blaydon and Koenraad Linder calculated the prevalence of exercise addiction among triathletes (at professional and amateur levels combined) to top 64 percent. (These cases, however, did not appear to co-occur with eating disorders, as few triathletes reported fears of fat gain or a preoccupation with curtailing caloric intake. Considering that the maintenance of a competitive edge in triathlons requires the average competitor to consume more than three thousand calories per day, this low rate of eating-related pathology makes sense: it would be nearly impossible to succeed as a triathlete without adequate fuel.)

As far as the amateur athlete or active community is concerned, many people may also choose to go heavier in the weight room (or harder on the track) if and when their schedules and other life obligations allow for it. As an example, a student on winter break may spend more hours in her hometown gym than she would during finals week at school because it feels good and proves to be fun. Absent pathology or compulsion, she still makes time for friends, family, and leisure activities. But once classes start up again she adjusts her gym schedule accordingly, perhaps cutting back on hours spent on the elliptical or switching the times of her workouts so she can complete assignments on pace with deadlines.

To truly discern whether an exercise regimen is pathological, what drives a person to pursue physical activity in the first place needs to be examined, as well as how that pursuit affects the rest of his or her life. If physical activities (or urges to engage in exercise-related behaviors) begin eating into one's relationships, work performance, sleep, emotional stability, and physical health, then what may have started out as a healthy pursuit has likely become harmful.

If, for example, the above student suffered from exercise addiction, she'd find it nearly impossible to relent on any increases in physical activity she may have introduced into her lifestyle during her vacation from school. Her growing devotion to the gym may begin whittling away the time she has outside of classes, encroaching upon her previous enjoyment of catching up with peers, her stamina for studying, or even her sleep habits. Her schoolwork may suffer as she forgoes trips to the library in favor of trips to the fitness center, obsessively clinging to an overzealous routine that leaves her exhausted and barely motivated to study for exams or spell-check assignments, let alone to take those brain breaks that help her recharge or grant her the mental ease to relax in the company of friends.

WHAT'S WEIGHT GOT TO DO WITH IT?

There's a debate among mental health professionals as to whether exercise addiction is its own, separate psychological issue or whether it's simply another iteration of an eating disorder. Individuals prone to self-esteem and body image issues who seek to keep their body fat percentages or total caloric intake at a minimum may utilize atypical amounts of exercise to keep their BMI down or to compensate for binges, effectively warding off guilt and anxiety associated with failing to control their size and shape.[10] If the relentless compulsion to exercise arises mainly in the service of weight control, the excessive pursuit of physical activity can be considered secondary exercise addiction.[11]

Compulsive exercise is a prominent feature of approximately 55 percent of eating disorders[12] and can be used not only as an alternative means of ridding oneself of unwanted calories, but also as a strategy to regulate affect.[13] Because eating disordered individuals are consumed by fears of losing control over how many calories they take in—the ultimate terror being, for many, an untamable weight gain that renders them "un-loveable"—compulsive physical activity may appeal to them in its dual promise to both compensate for nutritional indulgences and to accelerate metabolism in the interest of remaining inhumanly thin.[14] Severity of eating disorder symptoms is typically higher when exercise is relentlessly utilized as an additional means of manipulating weight.[15, 16, 17] Those whose eating disorders give rise to compulsive exercise[18] tend to suffer from more severe anxiety and nondiagnosable physiological problems (somatization) than those who struggle with caloric restriction or bingeing and purging alone.[19]

Primary exercise addiction, by contrast, does not have as its sole aim the burning of calories in order to control weight. Instead, an obsessive need to cycle through longer (or increasingly challenging) fitness routines ad nauseam, with strength, stamina, or constant motion as an end in itself, is primary exercise addiction's hallmark. Primary exercise addicts find a particular kind of comfort in the self-perpetuating repetitions they cycle through atop the achievement of that ever-elusive exercise "high," which boosts mood and dilutes anxiety, anger, and perhaps even the awareness of one's own vulnerability (or need).

Put simply: exercise itself is the gratification-inducing end in primary exercise addiction, whereas exercise is a means to another end (namely, weight or caloric control) in secondary exercise addiction.

Some psychologists differentiate between these separate manifestations of exercise addiction by administering a scale to apparent exercise addicts that measures their fear of fat (officially dubbed the Goldfarb Fear of Fat Scale[20]). Active folks who score high on levels of exercise dependence and low on fears of fat are grouped in the primary addiction category, while those who score high on both measures can be considered secondary addicts.

Irrespective of whether overzealous fitness pursuits are ends in and of themselves or arms of an underlying eating disorder, all exercise addicts are consumed to pathological levels by thoughts about working out as well as a restlessness that severely constrains their mental and physical well-being. Their attention to—and enjoyment of—work, family, school, and other non-exercise-related hobbies is encroached upon by the predominance of cravings to exercise along with anxiety in the face of missing an anticipated workout. What's more, their risk of injury (including burnout) is remarkably higher than moderately active individuals, and their overall quality of life is severely impaired by the time, stress, and isolation their disorder results in.

The relationship between eating disorders and exercise is somewhat complicated. Whereas most of us might assume that people struggling with eating disorders would do well to stay away from gyms or exercise classes—considering such individuals might be more inclined to utilize exercise in service of self-destructive attempts to restrict weight and calories—research suggests the opposite may be true. Studies[21] by psychologists at Kentucky University demonstrate that moderate, healthy amounts of physical activity may actually *reduce* eating disordered behavior and boost the well-being of those who battle issues surrounding food. Researchers believe this unanticipated effect has much to do with what the positive mental and physical consequences of exercise performed in moderation can confer. From improvements to self-esteem and body image, reductions in depression and anxiety, to increases in bone density, a kick-start to metabolism, and a healthy enhancement of musculature (read: strength), exercising within reason appears to mitigate many risk factors for eating disorders, watering down the severity of symptoms and improving overall mental and physical health.

Eating disordered individuals who go on to experience an addictive relationship with exercise appear to have been prone to do so prior to, or at the start of, their eating disorder. Put simply: exercise itself does not cause eating pathologies. (If anything, exercise in its healthiest form can ameliorate the severity of eating disorder symptoms.) But eating pathologies can and often do co-occur with unhealthy attitudes toward (and misuses of) exercise, especially when such behaviors are predicated on deeply rooted self-esteem, body image, and underlying emotional issues.

An individual's predisposition to dependency determines in large part whether hitting the gym staves off or encourages an addiction to exercise. The very behaviors shown to improve mental and physical pathologies for many may escalate all too quickly to unhealthy extremes by those prone to exercise addiction. We'll take a look at what constitutes this predisposition in chapter 4, "How It Begins."

3

WHO COINED IT?

A Brief History of Exercise Addiction

The symptoms of exercise addiction existed well before the terminology to identify them. Some theorists peg ancient Greece's national obsession with Olympian athleticism as the primordial breeding ground for pathological physical activity. "Addiction to gymnastic exercises of all kinds was characteristic of the Hellenic [Greek] people from the days of Homer," writes early-twentieth-century scholar Kenneth Freeman.[1] The athletes he describes appear to have been as isolated from daily life due to their adherence to sport as today's exercise addicts. "Competitors had to live in complete idleness from other pursuits," Freeman explains, noting as well the noticeable dependency many gymnasts seemed to develop on their sport of choice, such that a veritable state of withdrawal ensued in the event that they were prevented from training. "If they departed from their prescribed system of training in the very slightest degree, they were seized with serious diseases. Consequently, they were useless."

Concerns regarding the downside of too much physical activity date back just as far as the athletes Freeman describes. Plato and Aristotle warned of the threat that overly enthusiastic athleticism posed to man's intellect,[2] as did the fifth-century-BC poet-philosopher Xenophon of Kolophon.[3] Roman philosophers Cicero (a lawyer, politician, and Latin prose aficionado) and Seneca (the famed stoic and tutor of the Roman emperor Nero) further decried the predominance of training habits that trumped philosophic or scholarly pursuits, accusing overzealous sportsmen and their advocates of sidelining the mind and soul's superiority in favor of the body's cerebral vapidity.[4]

Though many prominent ancient thinkers considered fitness a marker of man's psycho-spiritual strength—the Greek poet Pindar, for one, composed lengthy odes to athletes, while Socrates asserted that "no citizen has any right to be an amateur in the matter of physical training"[5]—other critics went so far as to deem athleticism borderline malevolent. "Of all the countless evils in Greece, none is worse than the race of athletes," wrote Athenian tragedian Euripedes,[6] remarking that Olympian sportsmen are "slaves of their jaw and worshippers of their belly . . . honouring a useless pleasure."[7] The esteemed physician Galen of Pergamon, an advocate of more moderate exercise regimens that cultivated self-awareness atop bodily health,[8] concurred: "No other group of people is more miserable than athletes," Galen is said to have professed in the second century AD.[9]

Following the demise of the Roman Empire in AD 476, admonitions to cut back on exercise would take a hit—primarily because the ensuing political and economic chaos of the time left scant opportunity to indulge in superfluous bouts of movement (let alone focus on curtailing it). Amphitheaters and arenas in which athletes had previously trained were demolished by waves of northern European tribes,[10] and the Greco-Roman zeal previously channeled into sports was abruptly redirected toward religion.[11, 12]

Amid Catholicism's burgeoning influence, injunctions against pursuing bodily perfection gradually reignited across Europe as religious leaders expounded upon the potential contamination that honing one's physical strength posed to the human soul.[13, 14] During the Dark and Middle ages, sport would be reconceived primarily as a method to tamp down carnal urges as well as a means of practicing skills necessary for crusades and other medieval travails (e.g., jousting, equestrian aptitude, and wall scaling).[15] Leisure—not just sports, but theater and musical spectacles, as well—grew increasingly alienated from everyday life as the Christian ethic of hard work and labor assumed paramount importance under the influence of Benedictine priests.[16] Though tournaments and competitions hinging on strength and stamina persisted, church authorities tolerated them reluctantly.[17]

Anti-fitness attitudes eased during the Renaissance era, when humanism trickled back into intellectual circles in Europe. A renewed interest in Roman and Greek philosophies toward body and mind set the stage for reconsidering physical activity as a necessary component of man's well-being.[18] And beginning in the fifteenth century, sport and exercise made their way back into educational curricula.[19]

Despite resistance from religious circles that still considered indulgences in sport to be sinful,[20] physical education—in the form of fencing, ball games, wrestling, running, riding horses, and other team sports—gained developmental steam under the auspices of education reformers like Vittorino de Feltre and John Comenius.[21]

A renewed emphasis on the importance of exercise—especially as a critical ingredient in children's education—became particularly prominent in late-eighteenth-century Germany. Native teacher and writer Johann Basedow in 1774 founded the Philanthropinum,[22] an all-boys progressive educational school that interspersed three hours of leisure activities and two hours of manual labor (e.g., masonry and carpentry) into a standard daily academic program.[23] Olympic-style gymnastic exercises were also integrated into the institution's curriculum.[24] Basedow's Philanthropinum would ultimately fail, but his consideration of physical activity as an essential part of human advancement lived on through the lesson plans of numerous German educators who followed in his footsteps. Chief among them, Guts Muth, whose refinement of Basedow's methods eventually made their way to the United States several decades into the 1800s.

By the mid-nineteenth century educators and thinkers across Europe were sufficiently convinced of exercise's importance—so much so that several intellectuals began lobbying the Anglican Church to reconsider its staunch disapproval of bodily training. Making the case that physical stamina stood as a marker of man's moral fortitude, British authors Thomas Hughes and Charles Kingsley urged clergymen to advance robustness and masculinity among their adherents. Little by little, muscularity among churchgoers morphed from malevolent to meritorious as religious leaders became increasingly convinced that the corpulence and frailty of their congregations might indicate moral softness.

Across the Atlantic, an American Unitarian minister already concerned about the somatic shortcomings of his fellow clergymen caught wind of Hughes and Kingsley's agenda and set out to advocate for vigor and strength among churchgoers in New England, giving rise to what came to be called "Muscular Christianity" at the dawn of the new century.[25]

Athleticism's renewed prestige in developed nations across the globe didn't blossom without its critics, however. Some educators took issue with the newly standardized insistence upon sport in educational venues. Echoing the concerns of the ancients, one schoolmaster cautioned that excessive enthusiasm over sports risked eclipsing the average schoolboy's scholarly development. Describing overzealous adherence to sports in a language strikingly similar to modern descriptions of exercise addiction, Edward Lyttleton expounded upon excessive sport's potential to hook young, vulnerable men in a "subversive" spiral:

> A fascination, unimaginable by the outside world, urges him onward, and with a sense of his increasing importance, comes an increasing appreciation of the method [athleticism] by which he has risen; so that, even with his books before him, his mind is wandering among the scenes of his ephemeral triumphs and reverses [in sport] while he ruminates on his last big innings or the prospects of distinction in a coming foot-ball match. Prizes, places in the school, are but little things, and are treated as of little worth. This statement of the case is not a whit exaggerated as far as the majority of athletes are concerned. It needs a very exceptional boy indeed, after having been engaged in an absorbing pursuit, to unshackle straightway his energies and thoughts simply at the call of duty, probably uninviting, irksome duty. Under these conditions work, honest, spontaneous effort in other lines . . . is impossible.[26]

Within the same decade, rudimentary cases of what might qualify as secondary exercise addiction according to today's diagnostic standards for identifying pathological levels of physical activity began cropping up among young women—the majority of whom were institutionalized for eating disorders.

In 1874, Sir William Gull, an English physician credited with discovering anorexia nervosa,[27] underscored the prevalence of secondary exercise addiction symptoms displayed by patients under his supervision suffering from anorexia nervosa. Gull expressed astonishment about a "restless and active" patient of his remarking that "it seemed hardly possible that a body so wasted could undergo . . . exercise."[28] In 1892 another physician described a patient who was compelled to excessively lengthy walking "from morning to night, up and down the little garden of the house." The patient was also depicted as an obsessive player of "shuttlecock" (badminton) who would "[give] herself up to violent gymnastic exercises" when mandated by the nursing staff to remain in her room. "Even in bed," the doctor explained, "she goes on with her gambols and summersaults."[29] Decades later, the early-twentieth-century French psychologist Pierre Janet noted additional instances of potential exercise addiction among his own client population. One anorexic patient of his grappled with "a mania of walking of at least as great gravity as her mania of refusing to eat." Like today's exercise addicts who rail against the prospect of taking time off, Janet's patient exhibited immense angst in the face of reducing her time spent in motion: "If a limit is fixed of two hours' fast walking a day, she makes scenes about the calculation of the minutes,"[30] Janet wrote in a 1920 presentation on hysteria symptoms.

Back in the United States, the association between physical fitness and character strength, self-control, moral goodness, and the advance of nascent Progressive Era ideals was rapidly soaking up adherents. Fears of effeminacy among young men were rampant amid uncertainties about the American workforce's capacity to outproduce global competitors. Prominent educators fretted that weak men's inabilities to master mechanical innovations introduced during the Industrial Revolution would leave the United States in the dust of other developed nations racing toward technological prowess.[31] In homes across the nation, American sons were encouraged to hone their masculinity so as not to be labeled "sissies."

Yet despite the fervor surrounding fitness, it would again take second stage to economic, social, and political turmoil several years into the twentieth century. After the conclusion of World War I, families regrouping from its horrors weren't particularly keen on jumping back into militaristic fitness regimens. At least in the United States, more relaxed social activities—like tuning into newly popularized radio stations and seeking public entertainment—took precedence over most iterations of leisure-time physical activity.[32] Diluted by the shock of war and muted by the subsequent Great Depression, the pursuit of fitness in America seemed increasingly trivial. Not surprisingly, endorsement of physical activity and the accompanying strength of the Muscular Christianity movement waned.

Unfortunately, nonchalance toward maintaining the fortitude of one's body laid the groundwork for a relationship with exercise as misguided as overindulgence. Even as the economy recovered, most Americans held fast to their disinterest in being sufficiently active. This resulted in national embarrassment when a 1953 study conducted by New York University physical medicine professor Hans Kraus and fitness promoter Bonnie Prudden tested the physical stamina of children across the globe. Kids from Europe and America were asked to perform basic exercises—sit-ups, supine leg lifts, lower back crunches, and standing toe touches—in the interest of determining whether they measured up with the bare minimum medical standards for flexibility and strength. To the shame of U.S. citizens everywhere, 56 percent of American kids failed the tests. Meanwhile, their European counterparts flaunted a 92 percent success rate. [33]

In an attempt to rectify implications that American children were physically inferior—along with an attempt to respond to the growing body of research linking exercise with cardiovascular health—President Eisenhower spearheaded the Council on Youth Fitness, once again kick-starting the promotion of physical activity across the United States. (The vastly sedentary public was also shocked into more seriously considering exercise as a necessary health maintenance strategy following Eisenhower's own heart attack in 1955.) President Kennedy followed suit with his Council on Physical Fitness, as well as his own widely publicized personal exercise regimen.

But Americans' appetite for getting fit was most strenuously whetted by the fitness industry's innovations in marketing. Trumping government mandates and proof that keeping active might lower one's risk of heart attack, exercise professionals saw the powerful effect that marketing their trade as a means of promoting weight loss, status, and beauty had upon citizens' willingness to work out. Thus a newfound fondness for fitness began to catch steam amid cultural waves of "free love" and political tides of civil rights.

Jogging's popularity burgeoned in the 1970s, refueling the association between physical activity and moral superiority, while the 1980s welcomed a boom of health clubs and personalized training programs. Exercise's allure as an exclusive practice that promised to confer higher social standing upon its adherents was amplified by the redesign of gyms to replicate oases of luxury (think: chrome, mirrors, and carpeting) as well as the widespread celebrity sponsorship of training programs from Jack LaLanne and Charles Atlas to Jane Fonda and Elizabeth Arden. Compounding it all, fitness publications began storming newsstands across the country—*Self* magazine was launched in 1979, followed by *Shape* in 1981, alongside 1988's inauguration of *Men's Fitness* and *Men's Health*.[34]

Physical stamina was even overtly linked to Americans' abilities to lead, succeed, and be deemed professionally capable. Consider President Jimmy Carter's infamous fall while jogging a 10K at Camp David: detractors harped on this very human misstep to highlight his presidential incompetence. Or take Ronald Reagan's 1983 appearance on the cover of *Parade* curling his biceps in a T-shirt, just two years after he was nearly assassinated.[35] How better to communicate prowess, strength, and the capacity to withstand any and all professional challenges?

Whereas exercise in the nineteenth century had been a collective means of displaying national character indicating bravery and battle readiness, the twentieth century's growing fixation with fitness was distinguished by a noticeably individualistic streak. Health, in this more modern context, became a matter of personal responsibility and one's engagement in physical activity a marker of social capital.[36] Lifting, crunching, and jogging their way into the early 2000s, Americans reframed exercise as a lifestyle choice that rendered the "in shape" body as both personal enterprise and socially valid source of identity[37]—"a project and resource," writes sociologist Jennifer Smith Maguire, "to be managed and developed through self-work and market choices."[38]

Insights into the obsessive nature of some individuals' physical activity routines did, however, eventually catch up to the nation's newfound fitness frenzy. In 1970, a physician named Frederick Baekeland encountered an unanticipated difficulty in convincing habitual runners to reduce their exercise frequency for a study he was conducting on sleep quality. Few committed runners volunteered for the study, even refusing large sums of money offered as compensation. Those who bit the bullet and took time off reported astonishing dips in well-being—higher anxiety, impaired sex drive, restlessness, and interrupted sleep.

To better understand the phenomenon of withdrawal, as well as the pervasively heavy reluctance to take time off from working out, Baekeland[39] designed a questionnaire to assess his participants' degrees of suffering, unintentionally setting the diagnostic stage for preliminary conceptualizations of exercise addiction.

As research into substance abuse caught steam during the 1970s and 1980s—the National Institute on Alcohol Abuse and Alcoholism was founded,[40] the first "Criteria for the Diagnosis of Alcoholism" was published in the *American Journal of Psychiatry*,[41] and the Special Action Office for Drug Abuse Prevention was established[42]—so did the interest in applying addiction criteria to overly enthusiastic exercise. In 1979, sports psychologist William Morgan was the first to suggest that individuals who sidelined social and professional obligations in the interest of their jogging schedules might be considered addicts.[43] Ten years later, a British psychiatrist compared the behavior of overly enthusiastic runners with the clinical signs of dependence. On the heels of evidence confirming similarities between addicts' habits of drug or alcohol consumption and avidly active folks' adherence to working out—coupled with each cohort's psychological unease in the face of giving up their respective drugs of choice—epiphany ensued. Dr. David De Coverley Veale coined the term *exercise dependence*—namely, by swapping "exercise" with "alcohol" or "drugs" in an already established list of addiction symptoms.[44]

Research into exercise addiction has continued to grow well into the 2000s. More than one hundred studies to date have investigated the issue and there are approximately twenty-five measurement tools currently in place to assess the severity of overzealous exercise symptoms.

That said, research into exercise addiction hasn't been conducted without controversy. Some scientists[45] have challenged the disorder's validity by denying that an addictive relationship with physical activity could be truly unhealthy. (After all, they argue, aren't we more concerned about how many people *aren't* getting to the gym at all? And how much damage can be done through the activities that are supposed to improve well-being?) Others, like the authors of this book, have clamored to shed more light on the oft-overlooked physical and psychological dangers inherent in overzealous exercise[46] along with its pathological potential that places it on par with drug or alcohol abuse.

Though exercise addiction still awaits inclusion in the American Psychiatric Association's *Diagnostic and Statistic Manual of Mental Disorders*—as do many other behavioral addictions, which cause their sufferers to experience debilitating levels of dysfunction—many advances have been made toward better identifying its symptoms. Ongoing research continues to be conducted across the globe, and mental health professionals are becoming increasingly cognizant of an all-too-easy-to-mask issue that plagues a select segment of the population.

WHY DON'T MORE PEOPLE KNOW ABOUT IT?

Exercise addiction awareness has stalled primarily due to the minimal popular press it has received—especially when compared to the clarion calls we supposedly lazy Americans hear about getting off our butts and getting to a gym as soon as possible. The widespread promotion of fitness campaigns and health clubs has also emphatically drowned out attention about the possibility that exercisers might be using their regimens in self-destructive ways. While exercise addiction specialists have been fast at work seeking the origins and consequences of physical activity in overdrive—and attempting to communicate this to the general public—the fitness industry has muscled its way to pop culture's center stage, soaking up most of the media spotlight.

A look at the fitness industry's earnings during the past several decades hits home this discrepancy in popularity. By the 1990s, home exercise equipment sales had shot past the $1 billion mark,[47] steadily increasing from $54.7 million in 1980 to $1.79 billion a decade later.[48] During the same time, gym memberships flourished—jumping from eighteen million users in 1995 to more than twenty-two million in barely three years. By the end of the twentieth century, few could deny that fitness had become an important marker of personal, interpersonal, and even professional merit across America.

In 2005, 41.3 million Americans joined a gym. As of January 2012, more than fifty million people were estimated to hold memberships. (Whether they went consistently is another question: the International Health, Racquet and Sportsclub Association estimates that less than half of all gym members make adequate use of the facility to which they belong—i.e., going at least one hundred days each year.[49])

Growing encouragement from fitness professionals, exercise enthusiasts, and medical experts alike has transformed exercise into the next national panacea. With the obesity epidemic, pervasive cases of cardiovascular disease, diabetes, and other ills attributed to the much-maligned sedentary lifestyle, fitness has become a veritable mechanism not just to stave off physical health issues, but also a tool by which body-oriented individuals can heighten their social standing, demonstrate personal choice, and identify with a laudable leisure activity. (Small wonder it has become grist for addiction!)

Though a remarkable discrepancy exists between the fitness industry's cachet and the percentage of people who live up to its ever-multiplying standards—as of May 2013, the Centers for Disease Control and Prevention estimated that only 20 percent of American adults consistently meet minimal physical activity recommendations on a regular basis[50, 51]—the fitness and health club industries continue to rake in more than $75 billion[52] per year worldwide.

The United States and Canada generate the lion's share of the earnings—approximately $24.4 billion, with the United States alone generating $21.8 billion annually.[53] As of 2013, Britain's fitness industry dominated the European market with more than $6.2 billion in revenue.[54] Germany came in second, earning more than $5.3 billion[55] from gyms and personal training, while Italy came in third with $4.25 billion[56] in exercise-related profits. (Spain narrowly missed the top three European fitness industry competitors, coming in just under $4.2 billion.[57]) Latin America's 46,000[58] health clubs churned out $5.5 billion in 2013, while, according to the most recent reports from Asia-Pacific markets, Japan's $5.2 billion[59] in fitness industry profits trumped Australia's $1.8 billion.[60]

Examining the trajectory of exercise's dominance as a means of personal salvation from ancient Greece until today, a 2002 *Economist* article pegs the appeal of gym culture to its function as a substitute for religion.

> Perhaps hedonism is losing its lustre, and rich westerners once again crave the shape and strictures, however masochistic, that orthodox religion once supplied. Like Christian salvation, the holy grails of gym-goers may be distant and unattainable, and the paths towards them painful, but the rules and routines that their pursuit involves

seem to provide comfort to a new and growing breed of secular puritans.[61]

This quasi-religious zeal toward fitness is precisely what researchers and psychologists attempting to study or treat exercise addiction have come up against in their efforts. In the interest of educating the public about the risks inherent in clinging to the belief that exercise is a panacea, we hope to illustrate the severity of what happens when that which we unquestionably assume to be healthy turns out, upon closer examination, to be irrefutably harmful.

4

HOW IT BEGINS

The Origins of Exercise Addiction

Where does exercise addiction come from? Who is most at risk of developing it? And does biology or environment hold more sway in determining the severity of its symptoms? Whether you believe you might suffer from exercise addiction or whether you know someone who might have a problem, these are likely questions you've been mulling over.

Due to genetics, some of us are simply more likely than others to get hooked on particular behaviors or substances. Those of us who are prone to depression, anxiety, and neuroticism may be particularly susceptible to abusing a substance or overindulging in a particular behavior.[1] Folks who display symptoms of borderline and antisocial personality disorder as well as symptoms of schizophrenia are also at higher risks of addiction[2] along with sensation seekers, people who struggle with impulse control, and individuals who have a low tolerance for frustration and boredom.[3]

Brain regions that process pleasure and give rise to motivation and memory appear to be more sensitive to stress in individuals who suffer from addiction.[4] Additionally, addicts' brains appear to respond more eagerly to anticipated rewards, such as the high from a drug or the relief from a ritualistic behavior like repetitive hand washing or a daily five-mile run. This may be due in large part to a hyperreactive dopamine system in the brain—the neurochemical pathways that amplify the intensity of our emotions, that give rise to cravings, and that generate sensations of pleasure.[5] The more an addict seeks out his or her "drug" of choice (be this physical activity or chemical consumption), the more he or she reinforces that particular pattern of pursuit, rendering it harder to stop.

We favorably recall that which brings us pleasure as well as the route(s) we take to secure it. Most of us will continue to pursue a remembered reward in the interest of re-experiencing the happiness it granted us. As long as we can get on with the rest of our lives while seeking out that reward from time to time, we won't qualify as addicted. Trouble ensues, however, once we begin to prioritize the pursuit of that one reward above all other activities.[6] Addiction takes hold when we get to a point where we feel we *must* acquire a certain drug or engage in a particular behavior *in order to survive*. At this point, our brain chemistry may be altered from the repeated pursuit of our preferred drug of choice such that getting our fix trumps all other desires, interests, obligations, or drives.

A primary hallmark of addiction is its elusive promise to bring relief and pleasure through more than one avenue.[7] The behaviors or substances some of us become hooked on tend to offer us both a freedom from emotional or physical pain as well as a burst of euphoria. For those who choose exercise as their drug of choice, physical activity does precisely this.

Certain parts of our brain—such as the nucleus accumbens, anterior cingulate, forebrain, and amygdala—provide the neural groundwork for our subjective experiences of reward. We feel satisfied when an activity or substance tricks off just the right amount of excitement in these regions, and we're naturally inclined to seek out that reward again so as to rekindle such satisfaction. For many exercisers, ritualistic gym routines (not to mention the satisfying "wow, good for you" affirmations that follow the workouts) re-create those sought-after experiences of reward. To a brain that's genetically inclined toward addiction, achieving a happier state through physical activity may become fodder for compulsion. In the case of exercise addiction, brain-based reward systems may become hijacked by the obsessive repetition of aerobic or strength training activities, such that an addict's experience of pleasure becomes increasingly (and solely) reliant upon getting to the gym.

"I was fifteen when I joined my first gym," recalls one exercise addict. "At first, I seemed able to balance the time I spent training with the time I spent with my friends. But my regimens engulfed me at an astonishing pace. No sooner had I latched on to an obsession with burning at least four hundred calories on a specific elliptical machine than I had to add at least a half hour of weight lifting to my routine. I didn't see anything wrong with turning down invitations to social events to stay at the gym. I wasn't even concerned when I couldn't focus in class because all I'd be thinking about was how I'd work one muscle group one day and another the next. Exercise quickly became the primary source of my happiness, self-esteem, and sense of stability. I didn't realize until many years later, when I had an emotional meltdown upon learning I couldn't exercise due to an injury, how pathological my behavior had gotten."

Rewards, of course, encompass more than just enjoyable additions to the lives we already lead. In addition to procuring something we've long sought after (i.e., running a mile in less than seven minutes or seeing the emergence of our musculature in a mirror), positive affirmations ("you look *amazing!*"), winning competitions, or receiving tangible rewards (i.e., a prize for losing the most weight), the mere removal of something negative—anxiety, sadness, or physical pain, let's say—suffices to excite the satisfaction-seeking areas of our brains. The same pleasure response that occurs in our brains when we acquire something good (read: desirable) takes place with just as much force as when something bad (read: undesirable) is removed from our immediate vicinity. Psychologists refer to these different types of rewards respectively as positive and negative reinforcement.

Physical activity's potential to become addictive is heightened by its ability to both positively and negatively reinforce the exercise addict's behavior. Not only does it introduce pleasure into an individual's awareness by flooding the brain with endorphins, inducing euphoria and enhancing self-image and energy, but exercise also alleviates feelings of irritability, pain, depression, and anxiety, as well as self-consciousness and negative thoughts about one's body.

These physiological consequences of physical activity aren't innately pathological. In fact, they are precisely what enable many nonaddicted individuals to sustain healthy relationships with exercise. (As hard as those daily burns are, the anticipation of the exerciser's "high," the mental alertness, and the increase in body image keeps numerous active folks coming back for more.) In cases of exercise addiction, however, the balance of positive and negative reinforcement becomes skewed toward the latter: though the engagement in physical activity is still very much motivated by the pursuit of that exercise-induced euphoria and enhanced self-image (the positive reinforcement), for the exercise addict, remaining in motion is more about avoiding the consequences of withdrawal (i.e., guilt, anxiety, self-hatred—negative reinforcement). Working out gradually becomes the exercise addict's sole means of escaping emotional and physical pain, all the while introducing even more suffering into his or her life as the addict grows increasingly isolated, depleted, injured, and emotionally frazzled by an obsessive adhesion to an overly rigorous exercise regimen.

"Exercise was my escape—I would work out so I wouldn't have to sit with myself," recalls another exercise addict for whom physical activity was a means of "purging feelings of self-hate and keeping myself smaller," all the while granting her an intoxicating perception of being in control.

Sustained muscular exertion of all types alleviates a variety of negative feeling states such as anger, depression, stress, and even boredom. Boredom—especially the existential, my-life-lacks-a-purpose kind—is a particularly salient factor in the etiologies of all kinds of addiction. Everyone is prone to some degree of restlessness and lethargy, especially if our environments don't offer us engaging activities or enough entertainment. But those who are most vulnerable to addiction tend to be more easily bored than individuals who don't seem as at risk for chemical or behavioral dependencies. Circumventing the awareness that one's life has little meaning or purpose may therefore be as powerful a galvanizer toward behavioral and substance addictions as the neurochemical bliss they falsely promise.

"I honestly don't know what to do with myself if I don't spend at least two hours working out," said the first exercise addict mentioned earlier. "I think so much of my addiction stems from a terror of too much free time—of falling into some abyss of loneliness and purposelessness. I feel like I'm nothing if I don't work toward some goal of physical betterment every day. Even worse, I feel like I lose my sole means of organizing and structuring my day. Sometimes I wonder if I live for the stress my gym schedule introduces into my life—as if I'd be depressed by how unstimulating life might be in its absence."

In addition to the uptick in blood flow that wakes us up and helps us focus, exercise causes our brains to release a series of chemical messengers (neurotransmitters) that induce happier mind states and boost cognitive ability.[8, 9] Chief among these neurotransmitters[10] are serotonin, which helps regulate our moods; dopamine,[11] which pumps out in anticipation of pleasure and helps to regulate our motivation and impacts our attention; gamma-aminobutyric acid (GABA), which dials down anxiety and contributes to the perception of "liking"; as well as glutamate, which enhances our vigilance. Put simply, there's a physiological reason sweating it out helps take the edge off for anyone who gives it a go.

Lengthier exercise sessions also provide their own, unique "high"—a seemingly pain-free state brought about by our body's natural production of endorphins and endocannabinoids in response to extended bouts of movement.[12] Endorphins trigger feelings of well-being after their release from the central nervous system while endocannabinoids dampen our perception of pain. Running and other high-intensity aerobic activities[13] skyrocket the synthesis and release into the bloodstream of these neurochemicals, which achieve their psychological effects upon interacting with key neurological receptor sites in the brain. The end result? Similar to the consequences of ingesting certain drugs: euphoria, temporary relief from physical discomfort, reduced anxiety, greater feelings of peace and calm, a sense of "oneness" with one's body, elation, and transiently boosted self-esteem.[14, 15] Intense lifting or quick spurts of fast-paced cardio also have been shown to confer comparable psychological bliss via the same physiological mechanisms.[16, 17]

As long as someone works out in moderation—namely, by paying attention to bodily signals of fatigue or pain, taking enough time to recover, and making room in one's life for non-exercise-related activities—hitting the gym is a perfectly healthy behavior. Not to mention an ideal mechanism for coping with a variety of psychological and physical ills. Yet for individuals predisposed to addiction, such a healthy routine can get out of hand easily.

One study examining the brain waves of exercisers found that in comparison to active folks who displayed few, if any, symptoms of exercise addiction, those who scored the highest on measures of dependency displayed the most intense spikes in neural activity following forty-five minutes of sweat-inducing movement.[18] Such spikes in neural activity while engaging one's addictive behavior of choice mimic the elevations in brain waves observed in substance users viewing images of their preferred chemical.[19]

IT'S NOT JUST GENETICS

Predisposition, however, isn't the only factor determining whether or not we develop an addiction to exercise (or any other behavior or substance, for that matter). What happens to us as we grow up and foray into adulthood has an outstanding impact on how healthy or destructive our coping mechanisms become.

According to addiction specialist Durand F. Jacobs,[20] two crucial factors must be present in an individual's life in order for him or her to develop a full-blown addiction. On one hand, the individual must be naturally inclined toward excessive depression or excessive excitement—in other words, he or she must have a psychological bent toward chronic stress. On the other, he or she must emerge from childhood with deeply ingrained feelings of inadequacy, often due to severe rejection from parents or peers. With these biological and environmental stages set, it's often only a matter of time until the individual who inhabits them finds a behavior (or substance) that promises freedom from existential suffering. For some, drinking or drugs appear to offer a subjectively viable escape. For others, a rigorous fitness schedule that boosts physical stamina, introduces psychological peace, and improves physical appearance may appear as salvation.

The debilitating anxiety an exercise addict experiences when she cannot get to the gym as planned coupled with her preoccupation with planning the rest of her life around her routines reveals the contingency of her sense of self upon physical activity. For the exercise addict, to lose access to his gym schedule is to lose hold on the buoy that keeps his ego afloat.[21] Whatever the workout, to be hooked on physical activity is to be convinced that no other endeavor, save exercise, can offer the same sense of feeling okay, that obligations outside the gym merely get in the way of or risk barring access to the sole thing that renders one able to function. Repeating a preferred regimen day in and day out only serves to reinforce this belief and strengthen the exercise addict's dependency, amplifying the psychological consequences of taking time off.

Constant activity may also, for many exercise addicts, quell worries about never being good enough or, at the very least, distract from the existential preoccupation with worthlessness. As psychologist Claire Carrier[22] explains, "for certain sport perfectionists, the repetitive training, the body's addiction to movement, the ritualisation and the obsessive (but conscious) repetition of gestures . . . fill a vacuum of affection . . . to practice his or her specific gesture with no respite, to incessantly verify the mirror image and the image projected to others." Hitting the gym, Carrier continues, "revives infantile ideas of being all powerful" and "acts as a remedy for physical or psychological pain . . . in the same way as heroin does."

That a perfect physique is always just beyond the exercise addict's reach fuels the compulsion to keep working toward an ever-elusive goal, reinforcing the compulsivity of the behavior and ballooning the importance of being in shape or staying in motion.

In *Exercise and the Eating Disorders*,[23] psychiatrist Alayne Yates illuminates five different functions, ranging from healthy to pathological, that the exercise addict's obsessive pursuit of fitness fulfills: self-regulation, self-definition, defense against receptive pleasure, separation maintenance, and self-hurt.

Self-regulation entails the pursuit of being soothed, burning off stress, organizing one's emotions, or energizing one's body and mind. (The exercise addict develops a dependence on workout routines precisely because it boosts her mood, revitalizes her, and releases stress—at least at the beginning of her relationship with the gym.) There's nothing inherently pathological in self-regulation. Problems begin to arise when the gym becomes the *sole* method of self-regulation, such that non-exercise-related activities are ignored and injuries or illnesses are pushed past in order to achieve what the addict perceives to be homeostasis.

Self-definition is also a factor in both normal and pathological adherence to exercise schedules. Moderate exercisers enjoy identifying as someone who practices yoga, attends spinning classes, works with a trainer, or goes for a run several times a week. The exercise addict's identity, however, is predominately if not entirely dependent upon his maintenance of musculature, miles logged, or repetitions performed. He's come to believe his workout routine is him in entirety, and he reinforces that belief by sidelining most other activities so as to persevere in striving toward that ever-elusive fitness goal.

Defense against receptive pleasure encompasses the utter refusal to be taken care of, to relinquish control, and to indulge in pleasure. This component of obsessive physical activity is one of several indicators that exercise is being used in a pathological manner. Physical activity distracts exercise addicts from their terror of letting go, losing their honed physiques, or relaxing into the vulnerability of basic human need. Pleasure may be considered dangerous, tempting, a risk to the ascetic pursuit of perfection the exercise addict strives toward. Quality time with friends, family, and significant others is often considered by the exercise addict to be nonessential—secondary, that is to say, to the primary goal of success in mastering the body or doing enough to justify the fulfillment of needs (i.e., rest, hunger, or deriving enjoyment from entertainment). Consistently having an obligatory gym session to run off to, not being able (or willing) to make that dinner with pals as planned due to one's workout routine, or preventing oneself from catching up on lost sleep by setting the alarm early enough for that morning run keep the exercise addict in a perpetual cycle of obligations that crowd out any chance at easing into downtime.

Separation maintenance involves an addict's pathological need to separate him- or herself from others in order to pursue his or her addiction. All of us need some degree of separateness—privacy, if you will, or alone time—from others to maintain our own integrity. But as Yates points out, exercise addicts tend to push others away "to a pathological extreme," utilizing physical activity to "maintain such a pronounced degree of separateness that they appear inordinately independent."[24] Exercise addicts may frequently find themselves too exhausted to partake in social activities and family gatherings due to the rigor of their daily exertion.

"I plan my life around making sure I get a run in," remarks one exercise addict. Some days I push myself so hard that I have to drag myself through the day because I'm so tired. I'm often not present in my work, school, or social life because I'm either too depleted or I'm trying to plan my day to get a run in."

Self-hurt is arguably the strongest indicator of whether someone's zeal for physical activity has tipped into pathology. It arises when her chosen movements result in injury, illness, or acute pain that she refuses to acknowledge and chronically attempts to push past. Whereas an otherwise healthy exerciser would alter her routine, take an extended break from jogging or lifting, or reduce the frequency of the activity that's hurt her, the exercise addict persists. Sometimes the exerciser will adopt a new activity in response to an injury (mastering the elliptical machine, say, rather than running, or taking up cycling in place of yoga). Yet before she's recovered from her previous aches and pains, she's sacked with another injury after pursuing a new regimen with doubled or tripled intensity, likely a compensatory strategy to offset the guilt and anxiety associated with not being able to perform her former routine.

THE PERSONALITY FACTOR

A handful of personality factors appear to separate addicts from nonaddicts. Vulnerability to getting hooked on a behavior or substance tends to be affiliated with a higher propensity toward anxiety, irritability,[25] neuroticism,[26] impulsivity,[27] and irrationality,[28] along with a propensity toward harm avoidance, impaired self-concept,[29] and low agreeableness.[30]

The majority of individuals who develop an addictive zeal for exercise display similar traits. Like problem drinkers,[31] exercise addicts may be more naturally neurotic than those who can manage more balanced relationships with the gym. The hypersensitivity to stress mind-set of the neurotic (coupled with his or her rigid emotional coping skills) fuels compulsive pursuits of fitness, contributing to and feeding off of obsessive routines.[32] For the exercise addict who exhibits high levels of neuroticism, working out may be an attempt to quell the intolerable levels of emotional frenzy characteristic of this particular personality aspect—just as drinking or drugs offers a means of allaying mental chaos for substance abusers.

Neurotic individuals are also more likely than their emotionally even-keeled counterparts to worry excessively about appearance and health. Given fitness's promise to ameliorate corporeal deficits or prevent possible illness, exercise may be a particularly appealing behavior for the neurotic to develop a dependency on. Although the desire to improve appearance and health isn't pathological in and of itself, repeatedly hitting the gym out of neurosis renders an otherwise healthy pursuit dangerous. Since compulsions rarely cooperate with our body's warning signals—that is, *okay, I've spent enough time running, it's time to refuel*—obsessively striving toward physical perfection ends up threatening one's health in its relentless invitation of injury, exhaustion, and social isolation.

Extraverts, too, may be particularly inclined toward exercise addiction, considering they're naturally upbeat, energetic, and hungry for activity. For those whose energy levels surpass those of their peers, channeling such liveliness through working out may initially begin as a self-regulation strategy. If extraverts happen to have a constellation of genetic and environmental predispositions toward addiction (i.e., a heightened sensitivity to reward and low self-esteem), their coping strategy may be more likely to morph into self-abuse. While measuring the personality profiles of 390 American university students, Heather Hausenblas and Peter Giacobbi[33] found that those who displayed more severe exercise addiction symptoms also scored higher on extraversion than their less dependent peers. (Not surprisingly, there's a correlation between extraversion and substance abuse as well.[34])

Hausenblas and Giacobbi also found that agreeableness—or, rather, lack thereof—was an additional factor in predicting how likely students would be to hit the gym overeagerly. The less sympathetic, altruistic, and cooperative students were, the more intensely they appeared to be embroiled in symptoms of exercise addiction.

Competitiveness is a hallmark of less-agreeable folks' approaches to life, along with egocentrism, skepticism, and a propensity to flatter or deceive others for personal gain.[35] For exercise addicts, these characteristics may heighten an unquenchable urge to be faster, more flexible, more muscular, or leaner than fellow gym buddies; a haughty mistrust of professional advice to take off days or reduce one's activity levels; or a preoccupation with honing one's appearance so as to use it as a means of manipulating others.

Such traits of extraversion, neuroticism, and low agreeableness may contribute to exercise addicts' irrationality, irritability, and lack of impulse control—the very emotional displays they share with substance abusers and alcoholics.

CROSSING THE LINE—WHEN HEALTHY BECOMES HARMFUL

Exercise addiction can be incredibly tricky to sniff out. Many people misinterpret pathological levels of physical activity as evidence of an enviably superhuman enthusiasm. Regular gym-goers and even many personal trainers may notice individuals who stand out for their relentless adherence to cardio machines, aerobic classes, or weight rooms. Yet rather than being considered in need of help, such exercise zealots are congratulated, if not silently lauded, and used as an intimidating source of motivation by less fervent gym-goers. Passion, in other words, can often be the mask behind which pathology hides.

Appearances can also be incredibly deceptive. Although a higher body mass index (BMI is an indicator of body composition, based on a person's height and weight, that doctors use to estimate risks for weight-related health issues) has been linked to more anxiety about one's physique—which itself may prompt more aggressive pursuits to control one's size or shape through exercise—not all exercise addicts look alike. Some are prominently muscular; others, noticeably underweight, while many fall in between these two physical extremes. Several studies measuring exercise addiction symptoms and body composition, for instance, have found exercise addicts' BMIs to be relatively average,[36] clocking in at an average of 23.6. (According to the CDC, a BMI within the range of 18.5 to 24.9 is considered "normal."[37])

A healthy enthusiasm crosses into harmful territory when avid exercisers transition from using exercise primarily as a means of self-regulation and moderate self-definition to a means of compulsive avoidance of others atop an ascetic-like denial of basic human needs like rest, comfort, and relaxation—not to mention self-care and the pursuit of interests beyond the nearest fitness center.[38]

Picking up weights or pursuing cardio at a pathological level may look different than picking up a self-destructive drinking or drug habit, but the process by which someone becomes overly dependent upon physical activity mirrors the evolution of addiction to any behavior or substance.

A passion for exercise may develop as an individual finds relief from emotional or physical pain through physical activity, coupled with empowerment and surges in self-esteem. The alleviation of distress and

sense of euphoria derived from exercise is repeatedly sought as a preferred coping mechanism for managing life's ups and downs. The more
the exerciser seeks out the gym as a solution, the more it begins to
consume his or her life. Soon the initial twenty-minute elliptical session
that offered her a sense of mental clarity and calm must be doubled to
forty minutes to achieve the same effect. Perhaps cardio alone no longer suffices to quell anxiety and induce a better outlook. Soon, obligatory
strengthening exercises are tacked on out of concern that she's not
doing enough to control her shape or to stay in perpetual motion. At
this point, two or more hours of physical activity per day become her
norm. Off days are feared for the flood of negative emotions they tend
to bring about.

Once exercise has become involuntary or compulsive[39]—performed
to ward off or avoid the consequences of not cycling through the ritualistic behavior for fear of the emotional and physical turmoil abstention
brings about—the pursuit of physical activity has transitioned from pas-
sionately healthy to pathological.

When confronted by a friend or coworker about how the time she
spends at the gym is affecting other areas of her life (think: canceled
plans, absences from work, impaired performance on the job, or increased frustration with people she formerly considered good pals), the
addict refuses to consider her routine's negative impact.

She craves the gym like an addict craves the relief of a drink or a hit.
And in the event that someone else gets on *her* elliptical machine or *his*
Stairmaster during the specific time the addicts have allotted to work
out, they fly off the handle. He lies awake at night and finds his focus
dissolving during school or work as he ruminates about the next day's
workout, fretting that he may not have enough time to perform all the
exercises he feel he needs in order to function. Here again is a surefire
sign of addiction—when the body and brain adapt to the behavior or
substance, such that this behavior or substance is perceived as crucial to
survival.[40] In short, the exercise addict feels he or she cannot live without his or her preferred method of excessive movement.

He may be advised by a medical professional or trainer to take time
off to allow a shin splint to heal or a shoulder injury to mend itself only
to persist working out through the pain when he finds he cannot quit or
adjust his routines to allow for recovery.

The consequences of her obsessive regimen are ignored as securing her preferred fix via physical activity becomes her predominant concern. No matter the consequences to his emotional, professional, or social life outside the gym, he places his exercise routine above all other pursuits—if not to get that desired sense of euphoria and relief than to avoid the unease, irritability, sluggishness, and self-loathing he's learned to associate with *not* getting to the gym as planned.[41, 42]

According to the American Society of Addiction Medicine, "addiction is characterized by an inability to consistently abstain, impairment in behavioral control, craving, diminished recognition of significant problems with one's behaviors and interpersonal relationships, and a dysfunctional emotional response."[43]

For the exercise addict, the inability to consistently abstain manifests in the form of not taking time off to recover from injury or illness. Impaired behavioral control arises when the exercise addict promises herself she'll only work out for an hour and a half each day, only to find herself tacking on twenty or thirty extra minutes of movement at her intended stopping point. As for craving, the exercise addict thinks about his routine(s) constantly, sometimes lying awake at night or mentally checking out of work and social engagements to plan out his next gym session—or to fret about the consequences associated with not getting to the gym as planned.

Exercise addicts often fail to acknowledge the severity of their issues with the gym, expressing incredulity that their habits could be self-destructive (after all, *you're supposed to exercise regularly!*) or accusing those who raise concerns about their gym schedules of being misinformed and lazy.[44] The exercise addict's dysfunctional emotional response plays out in his excessive frustration in the face of a missed gym session or her utter disbelief and ire when another gym-goer interferes with her schedule by hopping on *her* machine.

5

WHAT IT DOES

The Short- and Long-term Health Risks
of Exercise Addiction

At this point, you might be thinking *sure, this exercise addiction thing sounds pretty awful, but if you're going to be addicted to anything, isn't exercise the best choice?*

There's a smidgeon of validity to that observation. Even the highest intensity running, spinning, and lifting routines won't put you at risk for, say, cirrhosis of the liver or the hepatitis (among other diseases) that alcohol and drug abuse can invite. That said, the toll exercise addiction can take is no innocuous matter. Abusing physical activity can wreak just about as much mental and physical havoc as a chemical dependency, damaging internal organs (most importantly, the heart and the brain) and harming muscles, joints, and bones. Add to this the detriment that overzealous pursuits of fitness can pose to people's social and professional lives, and the consequences of full-blown exercise addiction become anything but appealing.

ENERGY SYSTEMS

Even when we're lounging on a couch watching Netflix, our body is burning up energy. (Our heart, lungs, and other organs feed off our cellular power stores day in and day out, enabling us to function.) Just how much we expend at rest is dictated by our basal metabolic rate, which goes up or down depending on age, body composition, hormonal balance, how much we've eaten, and whether or not we've been to the gym lately. Partaking in any form of physical exertion, of course, requires even more energy—and when we recruit our muscles to lift heavy weights, sprint to catch a bus, or sweat on a spin bike for upward of thirty minutes, we really kick our metabolism into gear.

The calories we burn while exercising come from the conversion of carbohydrates, fats, and occasionally proteins into a chemical called adenosine triphosphate (ATP).[1] The bonds holding together the three phosphates comprising an ATP molecule contain energy—or the fuel our muscle cells use to contract. Each contraction is powered by the energy released from breaking apart the bonds between these phosphate molecules. And when we exercise, we're not only breaking down ATP molecules. We're also rapidly re-synthesizing them to sustain our movements.

Our muscle cells make anew or re-synthesize ATP either with the help of oxygen (aerobic respiration) or without oxygen's assistance (anaerobic respiration). Moderate- to low-intensity activities carried out over relatively long periods of time (brisk walking, a light session on an elliptical, or a reasonably paced jog) recruit the aerobic system, which breaks down fatty acids about ten to fifteen minutes into a sustained activity and transports them through our bloodstream from our body's fat stores into ATP molecules. This conversion process occurs in what you may recall from high school biology class as "the powerhouse" of each cell in our body: the mitochondria. And as you might expect, this process burns up quite a bit of energy, which is measured in calories (in other words: excess heat that is given off during the molecularly arduous task of ripping apart and reconfiguring ATP molecules to keep our bodies supplied with adequate energy). Oxygen is crucial in the aerobic process because it enables the complex molecular sequence responsible for generating ATP in the first place (the "electron transport chain") to function.

Fast-paced or high-intensity movements (i.e., power lifting or sprints) rely on the *an*aerobic system, meaning that ATP is produced in the absence of oxygen. This can happen one of two ways: first, by the breakdown of a molecule present in muscle cells called creatine phosphate (CP), and then by the conversion of stored carbohydrates (glycogen, which is housed in the liver). Rapid or highly strenuous activities require fuel faster than longer, endurance-based ones, and carbohydrates are a much quicker source of energy since they require less effort to break down than fat. Although the anaerobic route to ATP production is quicker, however, it produces fewer ATP molecules than its aerobic counterpart, hence heavy lifting and quick bursts of speed can't be carried out for very long.

The amount of time spent in motion without tiring is based on cardiovascular health and muscular strength and endurance. These markers determine how much oxygen is delivered to cells during exercise (the more those cells get, the longer they can churn out ATP for sustained fuel) and how much force a given group of muscle cells can generate.

Regardless of fitness levels, we all need to rest (at some point). Not only to allow our muscle cells to make up for lost ATP, but also to enable those muscle cells to heal from any and all damages incurred while in motion.[2] Each time we increase the weight, intensity, or duration of our workouts, our muscles incur mini tears, a natural response to the stress of exercise. This is why no trainer recommends repeating the same strenuous exercise several days in a row. (Muscle cells need at least twenty-four hours—sometimes forty-eight or more, depending on the strain they underwent—to build themselves back up again. Additional protein in the diet facilitates this recovery process, and some antioxidants, like vitamins C and E, are thought to offer muscles an additional recuperative boost.)

Our body is more than just muscle, of course, so our other parts also require downtime to get back into functional shape following a workout. Our brain, liver, kidneys, heart, lungs, and intestines need to recalibrate, as do our bones. Taking a day off from strenuous training is just as important to any gains we make in strength and endurance as the exercises we perform to make ourselves, better, faster, and stronger in the first place.

But many exercise addicts cannot conceive of taking time off from the gym—even if they intellectually grasp why a day of relaxation would, technically, benefit their muscles and organs. For exercise addicts, getting to the gym, hitting the pavement, or cycling through a lengthy cardio or weight training session frequently is perceived as a precursor to psychological calm, self-acceptance, and focus—regardless of how fatigued or overtrained their bodies may be. As we learned earlier, the exercise addict's avoidance of off days comes from a variety of fears, including the avoidance of withdrawal symptoms, an apprehension that not working out will precipitate a loss of identity, a terror of weight gain, or the overall black-and-white misconception that missed gym sessions equate with a dissolution of one's own value, purpose, control, and mental stability.

THE PHYSICAL TOLL

Joints and muscles are typically the first physical victims of exercise addiction. Sprains, strains, and muscle tears occur at a much higher rate among those who don't know when to quit at the gym. Bones are next. The risk for fractures, breaks, osteoporosis, or a lower-than-average bone mineral density (osteopenia) skyrockets when exercise addicts refuse to take necessary off days that would otherwise allow their bodies to recoup. Herniated disks, iliotibial band syndrome, tendinitis, fasciitis, and impingement are among other common overuse injuries about which chronic overexercisers often complain.[3]

Next come the internal organs. Recent research has accumulated evidence confirming links between overzealous physical activity and cardiovascular problems. One study on the cumulative effects of adding workouts to already physically demanding lifestyles found higher incidences of coronary disease among men who hit the gym hard on top of a workday spent performing manual labor.[4] Another study[5] found an alarmingly high rate of myocardial fibrosis among lifelong endurance athletes: half of the twelve subjects in the study who underwent cardiac magnetic resonance imaging displayed signs of a tricky-to-detect hardening of heart cells that, research suggests, may play a role in precipitating sudden cardiac arrest[6] or inducing an irregular heartbeat. And while runners who log between .15 and fifteen miles per week (a wide range, indeed!) benefit from an estimated 19 percent reduction in mortality rates, those who consistently surpass twenty-five weekly miles have a risk of death comparable to those who don't exercise at all.[7]

Among marathoners, the rate of sudden cardiac arrest while in motion ranges from about one in fifty thousand participants to one in two hundred thousand, depending on the demographics and age of the study participants.[8] One study comparing the heart's adverse response to marathons and half-marathons found that doubling the distance meant quadrupling the risk: roughly one in four hundred thousand half-marathoners were liable to experience cardiac arrest while more than one in one hundred thousand marathoners were at risk.[9] When patients diagnosed with coronary artery disease were split into two groups exercising at different lengths of time and intensities, those who worked out beyond the recommended sixty-minute maximum saw decreases in their antioxidant levels as well as a stiffening of their blood vessels.[10] Those who exerted themselves within a more reasonable range saw the opposite—a reduction in free radicals and improved circulation.

Imaging studies reveal that the demands placed upon avid exercisers' hearts—that is, more blood being pumped to muscles and brain—force their cardiac cells to adapt by growing thicker, stiffer,[11] and more voluminous.[12, 13] Compared to sedentary folks, lifelong marathoners have also been found to hold more plaque in their hearts.[14] In the general population, these physiological changes have been proven to promote atrial fibrillation,[15] embolic stroke, progressive heart failure,[16, 17] and coronary artery disease.[18]

Take a look at triathletes and the heart problems are even higher. One in every forty thousand college-age competitors dies due to cardiac complications while taking part in one arm of the multifaceted race. (Triathlons, which include running, biking, and swimming, range in mileage depending on their levels. The sprint distance triathlon mandates a .47-mile swim, a twelve-mile bike ride, and a 3.1-mile run, while the ultra distance triathlon entails a 2.4-mile swim, a 112-mile bike ride, and a full 26.2-mile run.)

This isn't to say that extensive physical activity is innately bad for the heart. Keep in mind that the above-mentioned rates of cardiac complications are low. But even the slightly elevated mortality rate associated with prolonged endurance exercise speaks to the heavy load that high-intensity activities place upon the heart. The greatest danger, then, seems to lie in not allowing the heart enough time to recover from exercise-induced stress. Exercise addicts who actively ignore bodily signals to rest—persisting in their workouts through pain and illness—thus may be placing their hearts in particularly hazardous conditions.

The kidneys also take a hit in response to extensive physical exertion. Though relatively rare, instances of acute kidney failure have been reported among long-distance runners.[19, 20] Scientists explain this adverse response to overexertion as arising from a spillage of myoglobin (a protein that carries oxygen to various tissues) from broken-down muscles into the bloodstream. The kidneys are primarily responsible for processing this excess myoglobin and when levels exceed a critical amount, the kidneys become overwhelmed and begin to shut down.[21]

Equally (if not more) sensitive to nonstop overexertion is the thyroid gland, which secretes hormones that help regulate growth and metabolism. Strenuous physical activity has been found to interfere with normal levels of circulating thyroid hormones in the bloodstream. In extreme cases of overexercise, thyroid function may become suppressed. Studies[22, 23] show this to be a more common occurrence in women than in men.

Lactic acidosis is yet another consequence of overzealous physical activity, caused by a buildup of lactic acid in the bloodstream at a pace that exceeds our tissues' ability to clear it.[24] (Lactic acid is a chemical by-product that our muscles and blood cells produce when they convert carbohydrates into energy. It's what causes us to feel the "burn" when we're lifting heavy weights, doing multiple reps, or running, swimming, or biking intensely. Typically, lactic acid buildup occurs during intense bouts of exercise, like power lifts or sprints, when oxygen is depleted and novel sources of cellular fuel must be tapped in order for us to carry on.[25])

Anyone who consistently overexerts him- or herself risks falling prey to overtraining. Higher resting heart rates, dips or spikes in blood pressure, dehydration, elevated body temperature, chest pain, irregular bowels and stomachaches, hampered breathing, changes in metabolism, and weight loss are among the key signs of overtraining. If left untreated, these physical symptoms can interfere with the body's immune response, chronically elevate the central nervous system's level of stress hormones, and induce anemia (a fatiguing reduction in the number of red blood cells coursing through the bloodstream).[26] The bodily duress brought about by excessive activity also prompts the brain's hormonal control centers to send "shut down" signals to male and female sex organs, halting reproductive processes in the interest of preserving what little reserves the overexerted person has left. When someone consistently burns more energy than he or she takes in—as can often be the case with exercise addiction—hormones critical to the reproductive process (i.e., gonadotropin-releasing hormone and luteinizing hormone) are inhibited by brain structures keen on sniffing out whether a newly conceived fetus can survive.[27] (Let's just say that creating another human isn't the body's top priority when it's being brutalized by too much time spent in exertion mode.)

For a woman, this means the menstrual cycle cuts itself short, markedly lowering (if not temporarily eliminating) her ability to conceive. When the abrupt stoppage of a woman's menstrual cycle accompanies osteoporosis and disordered eating, she suffers from what experts call the *female athlete triad*.[28, 29, 30] Over the long term, the female athlete triad has been linked to later-life osteoporosis and high risk for bone fracture, as well as for lower back and pelvic bone problems.[31] Whether the lack of menstruation due to energy deficits (read: too-low body fat percentages) locks female exercise addicts into long-term infertility is still under debate. Some research suggests that when women's weights return to viable levels, their menses follow suit and conception can occur with little complication.[32] Many scientists, however, caution that the medical field doesn't yet know enough about the long-term risk to fertility posed by a suspension in menstruation due to excessive activity.[33] One study that polled nearly two thousand female marathon runners found approximately 24 percent of them lacked a regular period while a whopping 10 percent were completely infertile.[34]

Even though most men remain technically fertile during times of heavy physical exertion, their sex hormones appear to be equally sensitive to the exhaustion factor of exercise addiction. Testosterone levels dip when they subject themselves to too much time at the gym, falling dramatically as tiredness from too much training ensues.[35] This doesn't even begin to account for the many health complications associated with steroid use among men looking to pack on superhuman amounts of muscle. Apart from lowered semen count and infertility, steroids can lead to erectile dysfunction; increased blood pressure; prostate enlargement and shrinkage of the testes; kidney, liver, and heart disease; and even the growth of breast tissue. Estimates of the prevalence of steroid use among men in developed nations across the globe range between 6.6[36] and 15 percent.[37]

Overtraining also alters its sufferers' psychological states. Weariness, apathy and depression, reduced appetite and fatigue, lowered motivation or vigor in day-to-day life, disturbed sleep, irritability, and impaired self-confidence are among the signs that a body's been forced to over-perform.[38] Anxiety is also a red flag indicating potential overexertion.

Whether a pathology undergirds their enthusiasm for sport or not, many athletes are at risk for overtraining—more than 15 percent[39] of all athletes are thought to be suffering from overtraining symptoms[40, 41] on any given Sunday, while more than 60 percent[42, 43] are expected to exhibit its manifestations at least once throughout their career. Add an underlying exercise addiction to the common occurrence of overtraining and its repercussions become even more severe. Whereas an athlete who doesn't have an addictive relationship with physical activity will take note of overtraining signs and cut back on her routines, an exercise addict will force herself to push through them, placing herself at a much higher risk of physical injury, mood destabilization, and long-term internal organ damage (reproductive capacity included).

When overzealous exercise is compounded by an accompanying eating disorder, the physical consequences are even worse. Consistently burning off more calories than you take in, restricting your food consumption no matter how much energy you expend, wreaks havoc on just about every aspect of the human body. Undernourishment throws off our balance of electrolytes, vitamins, and minerals; it interferes with our ability to synthesize hormones critical to metabolic and reproductive functioning; it encourages insomnia, impairs neuromuscular and cognitive functions (think: concentration, remembering which locker at the gym you left your phone in, where your body is in space), and it may irreversibly impair blood sugar and blood pressure, leading to fainting. Severe dehydration and chronic malnutrition can also take a massive toll on the thyroid gland, an endocrine organ crucial to regulating our metabolism and mood. The heart takes an equally severe hit when the body to which it belongs doesn't take in enough nourishment. Irregular heartbeats, poor circulation, and heart attacks are perhaps the most dangerous consequences of not eating enough. Additional effects of undereating include anemia, thinning of bones, peptic ulcers, tooth decay, brittle nails, hair loss, and the body's production of a furlike protective coating called lanugo. You might think that a person who religiously restricts his or her food intake wouldn't have the energy to get to the gym. But as many as 48 percent of all individuals suffering from eating disorders utilize exercise in an addictive manner.[44]

THE PSYCHOLOGICAL TOLL

As if the short- and long-term physical damage pathological amounts of physical activity bring about weren't enough, the psychological turmoil exercise addicts experience as a result of their over-the-top fitness pursuits is equally concerning. When gym-goers rely upon exercise to alleviate stress, they can easily fall into the trap of assuming that exercise is the *only* method to reduce anxieties and upsets. The more an exercise addict uses her fitness regimen as a means of coping with unwanted emotions (or excusing herself from uncomfortable social and professional situations), the more she reinforces her dependence upon physical activity, all the while whittling down her ability to function without it.

While going for a jog or hitting the weight rack is a viable and healthy method of stress reduction for a non-exercise addict, the increasingly rigid and time-consuming routines of the exercise addict often introduce even greater amounts of stress into his life. Guilt and irritability skyrocket when the compulsive exerciser must rearrange or reduce the amount of physical activity he'd hoped to perform.[45] On top of feeling overwhelmingly sluggish and fatigued on days he can't cycle through his workout, his vulnerable sense of self-worth that hinges on exercise starts to dwindle. Depression, helpless rage, and panic may swell to a hilt so intolerable that the exercise addict removes himself from all situations that threaten to impede his routine.

Consider the case of Ben Carter, an exercise addict from Australia, who ultimately lost a job and long-term girlfriend due to his excessive preoccupation with running, lifting, and obsessing about the calories he'd burned and the miles he'd logged each day. (You can read more of Ben's story in chapter 7.)

> If I was unable to work out or delayed, I would get all the classic symptoms of panic. I would be short of breath, have palpitations, and get shaky and dizzy. My thoughts would be racing: how can I get out of this situation and get my workout in? If I miss the workout, I will lose fitness, lose muscle mass, put on weight, lose all the gains I had worked so hard to achieve. If I skipped a workout, I was lazy, slothful, disgusting. I would be so disappointed in myself that I just couldn't sit with the feelings, and I always ended up giving in and working out anyway, no matter how horrible I felt about it. If anyone

got in my way of working out or if a friend or family member asked
me to do a favor when I had a run or session planned I just said no. I
was intolerant of anything that kept me from it.

The prickling frustration, intolerable guilt, and extreme physical and
emotional discomfort exercise addicts experience when prevented from
working out illustrates the intensity of their dependence upon fitness—
not just at the neurochemical level, as a means of reducing anxiety, but
also at the psychological level. Exercise addicts are often so wrapped up
in their workout schedules that they hinge most, if not all, of their
identity, self-acceptance, and self-esteem on how hard or long they
exert themselves.

A stand-up comedian from Boston describes her struggles thusly:

> When I was fifteen I started working out for three hours a day as part
> of a weight loss attempt. I would always keep adding and adding to
> my regimen, more weight, more reps, and sometimes more sets.
> Then the elliptical calorie count. I'd start at one hundred but each
> day I had to add a little more. At the height of it I was doing six
> hundred calories on the elliptical, three sets on every machine at the
> gym, and an hour of basketball. I stopped being okay with myself if I
> didn't get to the gym every day and do every move in my workout. I
> never missed a day, knew I'd feel like a piece of shit if I did. I
> organized my life around the gym.

For many addicts, chasing the illusion that one is "in control" of his or
her body becomes a prime motivator in refusing to cut back or compromise workouts.

"Certain parts of my life were out of my control," reflects another
exercise addict, "exercise and staying thin were something I could control so it became an obsession. I feel anxious when I don't get to exercise if I've planned on doing so—I feel lost and have a hard time being
present with whomever I'm with or wherever I am."

The obsessive craving and inability to focus or relax during non-
exercise-related endeavors that characterize exercise addiction is further compounded when an eating disorder fuels its compulsive cycle, as
C.—whose story you'll also read in chapter 7—reflects upon her secondary exercise addiction:

My relationship with overexercising began in high school. I noticed that running long distances changed my body. I was able to lose weight simply by being on the track team. But I just didn't feel like it was enough. So I asked my parents for a gym membership and started going in the mornings before school. I would wake up around 5:00 or 5:30 and run four to five miles on the treadmill at the gym. Then I would go to track practice and run more. Predictably, I lost more weight. But for some reason that I could not put my finger on, it still was not enough. I noticed a nagging voice that seemed to have effortlessly been ignited, whispering to me, "More. You need to do more. You need to be more." I began purging and cut down what I was eating even more. By freshman year of college I was struggling with a full-blown eating disorder. I was purging often, I was taking laxatives and diet pills—anything and everything that assisted in weight loss, I did it. The more emaciated I became, the less control I seemed to have over that voice. I began waking up at 4:00 am to run miles in the cold morning air. But it wasn't enough. Slowly I was losing grip on the ability to control my thought processes. I would wake myself up in a cold sweat in the middle of the nights, my mind screaming in anger at myself for having that spoonful of hot sauce before I went to sleep. I did not have the willpower or cognitive strength to talk back to that voice. Instead I threw on my gym clothes and darted outside for another run. When I got back I lay in my bed, sweating a cold, terrified sweat, continuously moving my legs and listening to the slick rasp of the sheets as I counted my movements in my head.

The chronic stress that relentless pursuit of physical activity puts on the exercise addict's body and mind amplifies her vulnerability to illness and injury. Chronic stress has long been associated with reductions in immune system functioning, heart disease, and depression.[46] Even if an exercise addict hasn't yet run into physical injury, her risk of long-term health consequences is increased by the unyielding anxiety, constant onslaught of stress hormones in the wake of physical exertion, irritability, and exhaustion affiliated with her compulsive reliance upon physical activity.

THE SOCIAL AND PROFESSIONAL TOLL

Exercise addicts' social and professional lives often take equally severe hits as their bodies and minds. Time spent in motion engulfs the majority of their days. The hours remaining after sweating it out, stretching, and showering after heavy workouts are barely enough for the addict to plan, refuel, and rest up for the next day's routine. "I quit what I'd once considered my *dream job* because I was too terrified of sitting at a desk all day," one exercise addict admits.

> I transitioned to a lower paying position at a health and fitness company primarily because they didn't mind how many gym breaks I took during the day. Eventually, I left that job to "freelance" just so that I could maintain my workouts while still getting enough sleep. My schedule while working was unmanageable. I would get up at 5:00 or 6:00 am each morning to burn *at least* four hundred calories on the elliptical machine, followed by a half hour of yoga, only to go back to the gym on my lunch break for an hour, and often for another hour or two after work.

The overzealous exerciser frequently dreads activities that don't involve physical exertion, given the anxiety-provoking impediment they pose to obsessively remaining in motion. Preferring the option of jumping into a jog or performing a sun salutation at any given moment, the exercise addict often opts out of events requiring him or her to remain seated for extended amounts of time.

"I lost friends because I only wanted to partake in activities that would involve some form of exercise," Ben describes. "If someone didn't want to go rock climbing, hiking, or cycling with me, I stopped hanging out with them. I justified this by saying we clearly had different value systems. But even when my active friends wanted to go to dinner or go to the movies I'd decline because I didn't like to be sitting for a long period of time."

In its full-blown form, exercise addiction walls off sufferers not only from friends, family, and coworkers, but also from experiencing pleasure, pursuing new opportunities, and most importantly, listening to their body's warning signals before injury and illness strike.

The tolls a compulsive relationship with exercise can take reach extensively into exercise addicts' interpersonal, professional, and emotional lives. Both their physical and mental well-being is compromised as they cling to a behavior in which they need increasingly greater amounts in order to function. At first glance one might consider exercise addiction to be among the "healthier" preoccupations upon which one could become dependent. But a closer look at the consequences of exercise addiction reveals that its health risks are just as dire as those affiliated with more "serious" addictions.

6

WHY IT HAPPENS

Thinspiration's Dark Side

So many of us consider exercise a panacea that we balk at the possibility that it could be used in a problematic way. Even close relatives and friends of exercise addicts find it difficult to take seriously their loved one's internal struggles. "Gee, I wish I could have some of that compulsive exercise," one recovering exercise addict's father often tells her, a response that's not the least bit uncommon nor the least bit helpful to someone trying to adopt a more moderate attitude toward fitness.

Wrenching oneself away from excess at the gym may be all the more difficult precisely because cultural attitudes toward physical activity are often skewed so strongly in favor of overkill.

"It's frustrating," says an exercise addict interviewed by CBS News,[1] "because here I would get my therapist telling me, 'Oh you gotta gain weight' and [then] I go to a gym and everyone's like, 'Oh, you're so thin I wanna be as thin as you.' It's like, well then why do I want to give this up? Everyone looks up to me, everyone praises me for how thin I am and how hard I work out. And then I just have this one person telling me to gain weight?"

The exercise addict is placed in a bind when her excessive relationship with working out gets in the way of social interaction, meaningful interpersonal connection, productivity at work, academic success, and even furthering romantic relationships. Yet her pursuit of fitness is perpetually reinforced not just by a misinterpretation of medical advice to be "more active," but also by peers and perfect strangers who laud—and occasionally express envy toward—her dedication to the gym.

Even if the praise one person offers another for his fitness efforts is subtle and unintended—*You ran for how many hours? Wow!*—the verbal applause conferred upon overly enthusiastic exercisers may interfere with their attention to physical limitations, especially if they're prone to addiction. Exercise addicts may be particularly influenced by encouragement for physical output. Not only might they be overzealously keen on chasing the euphoria gym sessions promise (not to mention the stress relief and anxiety reduction they often entail), but the sparks of self-esteem-boosting satisfaction that impressing others grants exercise addicts may feed their underlying need to bolster a potentially tenuous sense of self-worth.

HOW TOO MUCH BECOMES NOT ENOUGH

Psychologist Jim Orford likens addictions to excessive appetites: no matter the source of a person's above-average cravings, addiction diminishes his ability to moderate his behavior. Excessive appetites develop when activities that begin as pleasurable or rewarding (like eating, drug and alcohol consumption, gambling, sex, or exercise) evolve into necessities. You begin to *need* rather than to *want* an initially pleasurable experience, and a powerful desire to engage in your activity of choice progressively consumes more of your attention. Over time, the addict's primary motivation becomes the pursuit of that which he constantly craves—and he grows less concerned with the emotional, social, and physical tolls of his endeavor (broken relationships, loss of productivity, or decreased overall quality of life).

Such is the case for the exercise addict, whose initially healthy aspirations to be fit—reinforced by those gratifying post-workout "highs" and that warm glow of social approval—morph into an unbridled hunger for constant movement, a tireless effort to increase strength and endurance, and a fixation on body composition, calories burned, and time spent working out.

Human habits express themselves in varying degrees away from a norm. Whether reinforced by society or by the law (or often both), our actions typically conform to some mean or average. Those who display more extreme iterations of a given behavior are often labeled pathological—and they tend to be fewer in number than folks who display more typical behavior. So it goes, behavioral scientists[2] have argued for decades, when social control is at play.

In the absence of adequate social control, us humans lose a sense of what's normal. The result? We're all more likely to swing toward those pathologically extreme ends of behavior, setting the stage for more frequent (and substantial) surges in overindulgence. Or, as Orford puts it, "given unrestrained access to opportunities for appetitive consumption, most of us would be doing these things much more than we actually are."

Apply this logic to the growing number of exercise addicts across the United States and abroad and an alternative explanation for why folks are taking it too far becomes clear: in the absence of well-publicized and articulated upper limits to exercise, we really have little to go on when it comes to comprehending what moderation at the gym would look (or feel) like. Without effectively articulated limits and guidelines surrounding fitness and physical activity, the number of individuals for whom too much exercise is never enough can only be expected to grow.

Think about the last time you went to an exercise class that promised to get you in shape. Was the teacher encouraging you to tune into your body and slow down if need be? Or was the most repeated phrase during the fifty-plus minutes spent sweating a variation on "keep going," "don't stop," or "push harder"?

If meditating on the slogans that personal trainers and exercise instructors belt out with the well-intentioned interest of motivating clients isn't enough evidence of how moderation is rarely encouraged in the fitness world, just type "thinspiration" (or its close cousin, "fitspiration") into any Internet search engine to hit the point home. Take, for example, the following memes:

A thin woman squints in what appears to be physical agony as she hoists a dumbbell over her head. The caption: "If you aren't going all the way, why go at all?"[3]

A picture of a muscular man slumped over on a bench press. Caption: "Crawling is acceptable. Puking is acceptable. Tears are acceptable. Pain is acceptable. Quitting is unacceptable."[4]

A zoomed-out snapshot of a couple enjoying themselves on the beach, staring out at the water, doing "nothing." Caption: "Think of the consequences if you do nothing."[5]

Ominous pink and black all-caps text hovering over an empty, blurred room: "suffer the pain of working out or suffer the regret."[6]

The slogans slapped onto "thinspo" and "fitspo" photos and posters are illustrative of both the exercise addict's fundamental belief system as well as the fitness world's focus on disregarding bodily limits. The images these memes portray also raise the body image standards for women and men to a level that one body image researcher deems "far beyond what can be achieved with healthy or sensible levels of dieting or exercise."[7]

Though presumably intended as empowering, validating, or encouraging to individuals struggling to stay fit in an overly sedentary culture, the messages that thinspo and fitspo memes convey ring painfully true to individuals suffering from exercise addiction. While an individual who doesn't suffer from exercise addiction may delight in these affirmations and lean upon them as grist for working toward fitness goals—or simply laugh at their ludicrousness—the exercise addict identifies with their not-so-subtle implications all too well.

Take a closer look at what these taglines are truly saying: *you are essentially worthless if you don't work tirelessly toward some superhuman goal.* In other words, *if you cease pushing yourself, if you take a day off or rest, you will suffer.*

These are the types of dichotomous thoughts that characterize exercise addicts' internal dialogues, galvanizing them to ignore bodily warning signals, to push past pain, and to grow anxious at the mere thought of scaling back or relaxing on an off day. (They also echo the sentiments that fuel the exercise addict's avoidance of withdrawal symptoms— namely, the psychological angst, fatigue, and bodily tension experienced on the one day the exercise addict can't get to the gym as planned.)

From a metaphorical standpoint, the exercise addict may indeed be viewed as an embodiment of our society's all-or-nothing attitude toward fitness, as well as a reflection of our culture's competitive bent, tendency toward excess in the absence of boundaries, and reluctance to encourage moderation.

Although endorsement of physical activity and encouragement to keep going when our bodies (or minds) feel like giving up can be perfectly healthy sources of motivation for the vast majority of folks attempting to stay fit who aren't prone to overkill at the gym, their lack of emphasis on respecting bodily limits (in the interest of true fitness and sustainable health) may breed potentially hazardous appetites for excess. Those among us who are more susceptible to addiction, who are low on self-esteem, or who grapple with deep-seated body image issues may be particularly sensitized to thinspiration and fitspiration slogans, latching onto them as socially justifiable rationales to persist working out through injury, illness, fatigue, and depletion.

THE SELF-ESTEEM FACTOR

Self-esteem is the overall opinion we hold about ourselves based on how we were treated in childhood by parents and peers. It's relatively set by adulthood—perhaps, some psychologists argue, even as early as adolescence.[8] It's not very flexible, and it affects virtually everything we do—including the relationships we find ourselves in, our employment prospects, the likelihood we'll commit a crime, and our propensity to engage in risky sexual behavior.[9]

Low self-esteem has long been pegged by psychologists as a risk factor for addictions and eating disorders.[10] The less of it we have, the more likely we are to suffer from body image dissatisfaction and seek to manipulate our appearance toward airbrushed standards of physical perfection.[11, 12, 13] Those with low self-esteem are also less likely to relish accomplishments and more prone to taking negative feedback too stridently to heart. (One study[14] even found positive self-affirmations— i.e., *I'm great!*—can make folks with low self-esteem feel *worse*, inasmuch as they see all too clearly the discrepancy between how they're saying they feel and how they really feel about themselves.)

Exercise undoubtedly enhances self-esteem, primarily by improving body image.[15] (The rush of endorphins and social approval also doesn't hurt!) Yet the sense of approval, mood boost, and increase in self-image with which anyone who takes the time to be active[16] is already familiar may galvanize those at lower ends of the self-esteem and body dissatisfaction spectrum to start seeking it out excessively.

For individuals who have spent a great deal of their lives feeling disapproved of, unworthy, or unloved, the unmatched upshot in positive self-regard and social admiration that working out grants them may quickly become their most coveted pursuit. So much so that they begin ignoring myriad other endeavors, which could more enduringly bolster their mental well-being.

Whether exercise bolsters or deflates self-esteem seems to depend on the reasons a person engages in it. Those who hit the gym primarily to control their weight or look more attractive tend to feel worse about themselves over the long haul than those who pursue exercise as a means to improve mood, health, or general fitness (or simply because it feels good, is fun, and they genuinely like it).

Perpetually seeking validation via working out may reinforce the belief that one's value is predicated on what one can or cannot do at the gym. Tirelessly protecting their image through overly rigorous exercise schedules may keep exercise addicts locked inside a vortex of self-focus, disconnecting them from intimate relationships, meaningful activities, and openness to new experiences that would have a more lasting positive impact upon their happiness and self-worth.[17]

The exercise addict may fundamentally believe that he cannot achieve a sense of competence, connectedness, or support without going to the gym—nor might he believe that alternative avenues of meeting these basic human needs would equate to what he gets from his exercise schedule. He may use the gym as his main social outlet or as means of feeling superior to—and less vulnerable around—others.

Fueling exercise addicts' resistance to behavioral change is a hypervigilant focus on threats to their self-image, which is often enmeshed in exercise and contingent upon what they do or do not do at the gym. Whatever (and whoever) gets in the way of the workout regimens that transiently grant them a surge in self-esteem must be guarded against and avoided at all costs. This highly defensive attitude prevents the exercise addict from engaging in intimate relationships and participating in non-self-focused activities.

Unhinging self-esteem from external behaviors, like how much time one spends at the gym, is no easy task. But, as eating disorder specialist Lara Pence explains, "it begins with recognizing the parts of yourself you see as adequate—the character aspects people with low self-esteem tend to ignore because they're too focused on what they consider their flaws and inadequacies."

Pence works with her clients to differentiate false self-esteem from core confidence and to develop compassion for the qualities they identify as personal strengths. Rare is the client who isn't intelligent or talented in a field that's outside the realm of fitness. And often their exercise habits may be their main hindrance to success.

"Apart from positive affirmations, I try to go through a checklist with clients about what makes them feel good, what they would like to feel better about, and where they think they need improvement," Pence says. "Then we look at the evidence. Are they indeed good at the things they think they fail at? Rarely are they ever as bad at something as they believe themselves to be."

Without adequate self-esteem, we do not feel capable of taking risks, pursuing new opportunities, or even relating to others. For many exercise addicts, the gym has become their primary or sole means of feeling competent. The exercise addict expends so much mental and physical energy working out that he has little resources left over for alternative empowering experiences (being available for a friend or loved one who is having a hard day, for instance, or changing one's schedule to look after the kids so their partner can get a break).

In order to reorient themselves toward a healthier modus operandi, exercise addicts must learn to familiarize themselves with the assets they possess in domains outside of the gym. They must surmount the seemingly arduous task of abandoning contingencies as well as black-and-white thinking—that is, *I'm disgusting if I don't get to the gym every day; I will be less attractive if I cut my weight training regimen in half*; or, *if I don't get praise for putting so much into my workouts then I will feel worthless.*

If the exercise addict can adopt a learning-oriented approach toward situations that challenge his image or risk exposing him to those negative judgments from which he seeks umbrage via exercise, he can likely weather them more sturdily.[18] Such is the evidence-based advice offered by self-esteem researcher Jennifer Crocker, who has found that reframing experiences as opportunities to learn (about oneself or about others) rather than instances that make or break one's self-worth enables individuals to unhinge their self-esteem from external circumstances.

Another way to accrue a more durably positive sense of self or at least to find relief from the pain of chasing after it: take part in activities that draw attention away from your body, appearance, or fitness level. Think: learning a craft, volunteering for a cause whose mission hits close to home, or seeking opportunities to collaborate on engaging projects. "Goals focused on giving to others, or creating and contributing something larger than the self," writes Crocker, "facilitate keeping attention off the self and self-worth, and on a larger purpose."[19]

True self-esteem, psychologists Edward L. Deci and Richard M. Ryan[20] explain, is free from external circumstances—so you don't have to work tirelessly to protect it from constant threats. It's rooted in autonomy and self-compassion,[21] and it's the very stuff that enables us to be open to new opportunities and to remain aware of our needs.[22]

The ultimate boon to decreasing our reliance upon contingent behaviors that make us feel okay in our skin may lie in cultivating meaningful connections with others—a task that exercise addicts' gym schedules often make difficult. To truly trust that another person does care for or love her—indeed, to even allow herself to feel cared for or loved—can be an enormous challenge to many exercise addicts.

Over time and with the help of a trained mental health professional, however, exercise addicts can begin to internalize a sense of positive self-regard that inspires healthier behaviors, as well as tuning into (rather than ignoring) their needs. Sometimes, this may mean finding a new social group (perhaps even a support or self-help community) that provides the validation so desperately sought from the gym.

Exercise addicts may do well to ask themselves the following question: What do you let yourself do *after* your workout that you don't feel you can justify prior to exercising? For some, it's as simple as taking a shower. For others, it's curling up on the couch with a cup of tea and a book. Many exercise addicts also express a reluctance to be physically intimate with a partner prior to working out—oftentimes, due to a preoccupation with when they'll get to the gym in addition to how their bodies look without having already exercised.

Exercise addicts seeking moderation may want to try challenging themselves to perform these activities *prior to*—or in place of—working out. They can even be timed, so the exercise addict is reassured that she will not be engulfed entirely or cut loose from her regular schedule. The ultimate goal here would be to engage in these moments as fully and presently as possible for as long as they last.

Since exercise, like any behavior, is learned and reinforced by habit, unlearning the knee-jerk prioritization of the gym before all other activities is no small hurdle. But over time—and with the assistance of cognitive behavioral techniques that help exercise addicts challenge self-critical and obsessive thoughts or assumptions—a greater openness to, enjoyment of, and relaxation into alternative sources of satisfaction can be achieved. (For more on treatment options, please see chapter 8.)

This is undoubtedly far easier said than done. Old habits die hard and addictions may lose their parasitic life force even harder. Just like perfecting a new exercise routine or building a muscle, engagement with the world outside the gym takes practice for an exercise addict. It is the hope of any treatment professional dealing with clients suffering from exercise addiction—along with friends, family, and especially recovering exercise addicts themselves—that compassionate pathways toward self-esteem become less arduous for the recovering exercise addict. In the best of cases, exercise addicts come to experience healthier outlets as far more enjoyable, pleasurable, and rewarding than they could have anticipated when they were locked inside the shell of their self-destructive behaviors.

THE IDENTITY FACTOR

It's perfectly fine—and healthy, most would agree—to derive a sense of identity from carrying on an exercise-inclusive lifestyle. Calling oneself a biker, a runner, a yogi, or any other fitness-related label enables active individuals to differentiate themselves and define their uniqueness. It also serves to favorably influence others' impressions of them. Research shows that we automatically attribute positive qualities to people we're told are "physically active." Folks in one study who were asked to read about hypothetical characters who rode their bikes to work, regularly participated in exercise classes, or took sufficient advantage of gym memberships rated the individuals in question as more physically attractive, more confident, better at self-control, and more hardworking than characters who were described as less fitness oriented.[23]

Certainly there's no inherent harm in identifying with one or more modes of exercise. Those who aren't addicted to exercise can carry the socially laudable sheen of being "active individuals" while flexibly incorporating additional roles into their day-to-day lives. In addition to their workout schedules, they may attend PTA meetings or pick up the kids from school as a parent; get to work on time most days of the week and complete assignments within a reasonable time frame as an employee; carve out quality time to spend with their significant other as a boy-friend, girlfriend, or spouse; participate in a book club as an avid reader; or attend a cooking class as a self-identified foodie. Physical activity may be important to their identities, but it is not the be-all and end-all of their existence. Where problems arise is when exercise becomes the *only* activity from which a person draws his or her sense of self—and especially when the pursuit of fitness gets in the way of developing interest in non-exercise-related endeavors.

Because physical activity consumes such a large part of exercise ad-dicts' lives, most find little (if any) time to take on professional and personal responsibilities outside the gym—or to pursue hobbies that don't involve donning their sweatpants. The prioritization of working out above all else eats into more than just their availability. Exercise addicts' stamina, focus, motivation, and patience are typically strained, leaving them little mental and physical energy to devote to time-con-suming or stressful tasks. For many addicts, even if they're exhausted from not taking adequate time to recover, a large part of their aware-ness may be devoted to planning their next workout. This can impinge greatly on their ability to be fully present in meetings and classes or when spending time with a friend or family member and even being intimate with a partner.

"At the height of my exercise addiction," one addict recalls, "I was barely able to focus during brainstorming sessions at the magazine I once worked at. I couldn't stop worrying about whether I'd done *enough* stretching after my workout and whether I'd be able to finish up where I left off in my weight-training routine at lunch break before an afternoon assignment was due. I just felt so disconnected, so preoccu-pied with anxiety when I wasn't at the gym."

Many exercise addicts also express a destabilizing unfamiliarity with whom they are outside their workout regimens. "It got to the point where I didn't even have a sense of what movies or music I liked," recalls Kaila Prins, whose story you'll read in our next chapter. "I had no identity outside my exercise program."

Even finding a style of clothing to wear can be challenging, as some exercise addicts equate non-workout-friendly garb with entrapment. "I literally felt like I was in shackles when I wore anything other than spandex," another exercise addict reflects. "Jeans, office attire, getting dressed up—I never understood how other people could feel good in clothes that restricted their movement or made them walk slower."

AVOIDANCE OF INTIMACY AND PLEASURE

What else might account for the seemingly inhuman zeal the exercise addict develops toward physical activity? According to some theorists, an enormous motivator to remain in motion as often and intensely as possible boils down to a terror of intimacy—and a continual effort not to appear, or perceive oneself, as vulnerable.

"Obligatory runners," writes Alayne Yates, "are extremely uncomfortable when they are in a position of taking in or receiving pleasure."[24] Not just the behavior of exercise, but also the excessive focus on when they can next jump into motion may enable exercise addicts to distance themselves from feeling, being aware of their needs, and taking the risk of relying upon others to get those needs met.

"They maintain such a pronounced degree of separateness that they appear inordinately independent," writes Yates. "Many of them manage to avoid all close relationships through their dogged adherence to exercise."[25]

Illustrating the desire to keep relaxation and pleasure at bay lest it prevent the obligatory exerciser from maintaining control over his body and caloric output, Yates challenges the motives behind the compulsory early morning run: "Does the runner 'hit the road' at 5:00 am to be alone and self-reflective or to avoid the pleasures of sleeping late?"

The goal of constant activity may be, in large part, distraction from the sense that one is inferior, defective, weak, or otherwise "unacceptable." Yates describes how the average exercise addict "oscillates between the dangers of hunger, exhaustion, or external circumstance; the struggle to maintain a separate state; and the fantasy or triumph over the body. The oscillation generates excitement, and the excitement defends against the anxiety of being overwhelmed by neediness."[26]

A preoccupation with activity, independence, and ostensible self-control may protect the exercise addict from acknowledging her own human shortcomings (including the need to be taken care of). Keeping her focus on constant activity, haranguing herself when she isn't able to run as fast or lift as hard as she did on a previous day, and isolating herself with a repetitive cycle of endless workouts may also serve as a means of suppressing the denied desire to "be caught, restrained, and ultimately cared for." It is also possible that many exercise addicts may be motivated to drive themselves to injury or illness so as to be prevented from obsessively pushing their bodies past emotional and physical limits. As Yates observes, those who continuously overexercise "may wish that they would be apprehended so that they could escape the activity which controls their thoughts and actions. In this manner they could back into receptive pleasure—forced into having their needs fulfilled, though they may continue to resist every inch of the way."[27]

That toiling away on the treadmill, trail, bike, pool, or yoga mat (yes, unfortunately some folks even overdo asanas!) will eventually force him to suspend his relentless routine may appeal to the exercise addict's repressed yearning to be taken care of, to ask for help, or to justify forgoing the pressure to be perpetually active so as to (finally) rest.

REELING IT IN

Per Orford, the main way to encourage moderation among "appetitive behaviors" (again, any activity that affords us pleasure and reward or that fulfills real or perceived needs) is to introduce deterrents to their excess. These can be social, legal, or biological in nature and serve to constrict behavioral extremes to statistical minorities (the tails of a bell curve, so to speak).

Rare is the person who sees another's problematic consumption of drugs or alcohol and remarks, "Keep going!"; "I wish I could be like you!"; or "You look *great!*" Yet many individuals who witness an exercise addict's overzealous habits—think: running despite injury or illness, never taking a day off, succumbing to anxiety when faced with the prospect of missing a gym session, or appearing visibly exhausted from daily morning runs or lunch-hour power workouts—encourage a pathological behavior by expressing awe, amazement, or even mock envy at an exercise addict's seemingly inhuman feats.

Fitness professionals and gym-goers who haven't been educated about the consequences of exercise addiction—and the oft-overlooked necessity of moderation in physical activity—often support unhealthy attitudes toward exercise without intending any harm at all. ("Wow! Three-and-a-half hours today? I'm so jealous." "You must be exhausted. But I admire your drive!")

Exercise addiction is not on most of our radars. Why would it be when more than 46 percent of the American population struggled to meet the minimal amount of recommended weekly physical activity in 2012?[28] Unlike drug, alcohol, or gambling addictions, there are virtually no social or legal constraints upon exercise behavior that would draw awareness to its potential for harm. Considering the widespread concern with our nation's obesity epidemic, worries over people exercising too much have been relatively silenced.

By no means should physical activity be legally limited or criminalized. Certainly the last thing the general public needs to hear is a warning to stay away from picking up a pair of weights or to avoid trying to fit a few light aerobic activities into their lifestyles. But burgeoning misinformed fitness advice that convinces us to ignore our bodily needs (including our stress levels) and push ourselves far beyond our human limits to achieve unnaturally thin or muscular ideals has prompted a need for greater awareness among active individuals about limits, moderation, and the risks of overzealous exercise behavior.

It is our hope, in writing this book, that more attention will be paid to the small but potentially growing population that suffers from exercise addiction. As fitness wends its way deeper into our culture, we hope enthusiasts can remain cognizant of the disorder's signs and sensitive to the ways in which motivational advice may fuel unhealthy habits.

SOLUTIONS?

Gyms don't yet follow the lead of gambling facilities or bars by posting hotline numbers for folks to call if they think they have a problem with a particular behavior. But some mental health advocates are paving the way for fitness professionals to at least learn how to better recognize, address, and work with clients who present symptoms of exercise addiction.

Among these leaders are Jodi Rubin, who has designed a course for fitness professionals called "Destructively Fit," which explains the etiology of eating disorders and pathological uses of exercise and offers advice on how to approach clients who may have a problem. Rubin's program counts toward continuing education credits for trainers and instructors affiliated with National Academy of Sports Medicine (NASM) and American Council on Exercise (ACE) and is listed in our resources section.

The National Eating Disorders Association also offers a tool kit for coaches and trainers working in high schools or colleges that offers guidance on how to identify unhealthy uses of sport among students. Coaches can often find themselves at the forefront of enabling athletes struggling with symptoms of exercise addiction to recognize they have a problem.

One of the most difficult hurdles encountered by those close to an exercise addict is the latter's refusal to admit that his or her habits are in any way detrimental. To even remotely consider the idea that their relationship to exercise borders on unhealthy, exercise addicts must not only have a close connection with the individuals who confront them, but also must trust their authority and expertise. Coaches are in a prime position to break the ice, given not just their familiarity and knowledge of sport, exercise, and the body, but their ability to sniff out signs of fatigue, excessive weight loss, or anxiety.

Those who themselves aren't versed in fitness may risk further alienating loved ones they believe suffer from exercise addiction when confronting them, as the exercise addict may be more inclined to attribute their concerns to ignorance surrounding physical activity or a lack of understanding about why or how much one should work out. (For more advice on how to approach or confront someone you think may suffer from exercise addiction, please read chapter 9, "How to Approach Someone with a Problem.")

The American College of Sports Medicine offers advice about detecting athletes who may be using exercise as an alternative means of purging, along with several resources illustrating the prevalence and risk of excessive physical activity. Intriguingly, the only mention of "exercise addiction"—in a 2011 press release that read in part "exercise 'addiction' (the healthy kind!)"—on their publicly accessible Web site illustrates the pervasive misconception that an addiction to the gym is inherently healthy.[29]

Mention of the risks inherent in abusing fitness is also lacking on the President's Council on Fitness, Sports, and Nutrition—though the U.S. Department of Health and Human Services devotes a thorough chapter of its Physical Activity Guidelines to safety and the avoidance of injury while working out.[30]

Although we hear about guidelines regarding length of cardio sessions or number of weight-lifting repetitions, surpassing those thirty minutes or three sets rarely incurs disapproval. Fitness professionals must be attentive to communicating the importance of moderation to their clients, as much as they challenge their clients to improve strength, flexibility, endurance, or agility.

Health clubs may do well to offer resources to those who find themselves slipping into the throes of exercise addiction. The fact that there are virtually no lifelines offered to gym-goers grappling with exercise addiction symptoms may render fitness centers as catalysts for the disorder's spread.

EXCESS ADDS UP

When comparing exercise addiction to other mental health problems like substance disorders or behavioral addictions, most of us assume the societal toll would be comparatively slim. But the Centers for Disease Control and Prevention estimates that at least 2,117,000 people were admitted to emergency rooms across the United States for sprains and strains due to overexertion in 2010.[31] Multiply that by the average cost of an emergency room visit—$1,233 as of 2013[32]—and the consequences of overzealous or improper physical activity amounts to well over $2 billion ($2,610,261,000 to be precise).

That's not even considering the fifty thousand people[33] who seek emergency care each year due to fitness equipment mishaps at the gym (add $61,650,000—lawsuits not included), the five hundred thousand or so cyclists[34] annually rushed to hospitals after crashes (add $616,500,000), nor the eleven million Americans who suffer from eating disorders[35]—48 percent of whom exercise excessively[36] to control weight—and cost the United States $271 million in hospital bills as of 2006.[37]

That's enough to top $3.5 billion.

What's more, an average of 25.9 recreational exercise-related injuries are thought to occur per 1,000 people[38] in the United States, prompting 28 percent of working adults to take time off work to recover.

An estimated 970,801 weight-training related injuries cropped up between 1990 and 2007.[39] And among marathon runners tracked for a year and a half, 85 percent suffered *at least* one training-related injury[40]—evening out to a whopping 159 injuries per every 100 runners each year.

Sixteen percent of active men and 14 percent of active women whose exercise habits were tracked for a year[41] reported injuries related to their aerobic pursuits (from running and biking to swimming and racquet sports). And among athletes, traumatic brain injuries (TBIs) have been dramatically rising during the past decade[42]—a 2006 report[43] estimated the prevalence of sports-related TBIs to fall between 1.6 and 3.8 million per year.

In addition to medical bills, lost productivity at work, and emotional stress brought about by exercise in overdrive, the damage that out-of-control activity can wreak upon exercise addicts' bodies may have an additional dire consequence. Chronic overexertion—or even a severe, one-time injury—may render some exercise addicts physically incapable of maintaining a regular exercise regimen throughout their life spans.

Because they are more likely than moderately active folks to suffer wears, tears, sprains, strains, and breaks (not to mention bone density and metabolic complications), they may be rendering their bodies physically incapable of sustaining normal amounts of exercise well into old age.

Especially if malnutrition accompanies overzealous physical activity, osteoporosis and arthritis may force exercise addicts to reduce their gym time to minimal levels, further diminishing their morale, physical health, and mental well-being in the long run.

There's also much to be said about the expenses gym memberships, athletic wear, and sports-related nutrition that exercise addicts (and their families) accrue. In 2012, American health clubs raked in more than $25 million. Yoga and pilates studios earned just under $7 million, and personal trainers alone cost Americans more than $7 million.

Money spent on fitness apparel is projected to top $180 billion by 2018[44] while the Fitness Nutrition Food and Sports Drink sector trails behind at an estimated $55 billion.

Clearly, the costs of exercise addiction can add up. Although spending money on health and self-care is an inevitable part of everyone's lives, exercise addicts, in addition to diminishing their bodies and minds, risk watching their bank accounts suffer the same depletion as their overall health.

7

WHAT IT FEELS LIKE

Exercise Addicts' True Stories

KATHERINE SCHREIBER

The moment I became cognizant of my body I wanted to change it. Perhaps the bounds of my self-concept were too porous to keep out my culture's insistence on feminine thinness and the campaigns of the 1990s to wage war against bodies in their natural state by obligatory exercise coupled with caloric restriction.

Perhaps I internalized the anxieties of my mother, a chronic dieter who continually struggled with her own weight, compounded by my father's disapproval of her naturally expanded form after she gave birth to me.

Some girls are buffered from the self-esteem blows brought about by comparing ourselves to airbrushed models and hearing about how much less we should be eating by a strong family structure, a supportive school system, and a solid group of friends. I'm not sure my moorings were that stable, looking back on it all. As early as kindergarten I was convinced I was physically defective in a way other girls were not.

I wanted to be pretty like them. Quieter. Shy. The less conspicuous, the better, I thought. Meek girls got more attention and praise. Loud, boisterous, tomboyish ones like me who eschewed dresses and skirts and opted to wrestle with boys rather than play princess were told to pipe down and sit still.

I was always incredibly active. Hyperactive, teachers called me, once elementary school began. Too energetic for a girl. Too competitive in gym class. Too restless during reading time. In short: too much to handle. By the time I reached middle school, enough authority figures had chided me for the aggressiveness of my personality that I knew I had to do something to make myself smaller—in order to be an acceptable girl, that is.

Strangely enough, what I'd call my body image struggles began with attempts to *put on* weight so as to have breasts and a rounder face like the rest of the girls in my junior high class. (I was a late bloomer: an additional confirmation, I assumed, of the unacceptable weirdness that precluded me from any legitimate access to the legions of popular females in my class.) I was jealous of other girls' soft edges and mounds of flesh where I was flat, angled, and anything but smooth. I was scabbed and calloused from sports (soccer was my extracurricular sanctuary and gym class was my in-school saving grace). Most days, I excused myself from classes to hide in the girls' bathroom with a turtleneck sweater pulled up over my face, begging teachers who implored me to return to let me be because I was "too ugly" to be seen by other students.

A student a few years older than me came in during one of my episodes and deduced, from a project she was working on in social studies, that I fit the bill for body dysmorphic disorder. I told her that didn't make me feel any better and resolved to remain on the green tiled floor until recess—where, at the very least, I could try beating a boy in sprints across our school's terrace.

I resolved to quit sports and start eating as much as possible in the hopes that this would materialize a valid reason for me to shop for a bra. It worked eventually, and by the time my weight got up to a level that some doctors warned was "chubby," there were more than a few additional concerns on my proverbial plate.

The day I began my first year of eighth grade in a private school on Manhattan's Upper West Side, two airplanes tore through the bellies of the Twin Towers, eighty city blocks south. I'd come back to school from a summer clipped by the news that my parents were getting a divorce and I was already reeling from the hole in my home left by my father's abrupt absence. Everywhere around me, the world was falling apart. I could barely control my own body, let alone the environment in which it existed.

Rather than standing tall and seeking refuge through school, I predicated the survival of my identity upon blue hair, black lipstick, and death metal, and I hurled myself toward procuring whatever illegal substances I could find. (You'd be surprised how much a thirteen-year-old in New York City can get her hands on.) Physical activity all but ceased by summertime, and by the first month of ninth grade my parents agreed I needed serious help.

In 2002 I was forcibly enrolled in a nine-week adolescent boot camp program in Naples, Idaho, followed by a seven-month stint in a residential treatment facility for "troubled girls" in Bethlehem, Connecticut. It was in the latter location that the roots of my eating disorder and pathological relationship to physical activity would truly take hold.

Living among other emotionally disturbed women, I swiftly picked up on the maniacal race to be the thinnest, most troubled resident at the table. (Strange how even sickness can be a source of competition among women.) I knew that to win I needed to sneak off to my room and do crunches, jumping jacks, anything to raise my heart rate for the allotted forty-five minutes during which I was allowed to be alone.

Though I graduated from the program still at a moderately healthy weight, the insatiable urge to truncate my size had been set. As I transitioned back to my former high school—under the strict promise that if I got anything less than a B average I'd be sent away again—I clung to the meaning that striving to be fitter gave to my painfully self-conscious existence.

I succeeded in my courses and surpassed the expectations of teachers who'd cautioned I might not be fit for the school given my previous behavior, all the while chasing freedom from concerns that I wasn't in absolute control of my body by restricting my food intake and doing as many crunches, squats, and burpees as I possibly could.

When my school's gym closed down for renovations later that year, the administration brokered a deal with our local sports club that enabled students to use its facilities as a substitute for P.E. class. Thus I was introduced to one of the most ravenous loves of my life: the elliptical machine. (Yes, that may sound ridiculous. But it was, and still is, true.)

No validation was greater than the delicious confirmation that I'd burned upward of two hundred calories in a single, twenty-minute session bought on a device that didn't judge me, didn't fall apart, and was always, reliably, in the same place on the second floor of the cardio section. Here was a relationship I could trust, I began to realize—a ritual that made me feel safer, acceptable, accomplished.

It didn't take long before two hundred doubled, then tripled, along with the introduction of weight training, flexibility work, and an obsessive goal to have a six-pack by the school year's end. I cut back my food intake to facilitate the process and dropped weight rapidly during the spring semester. Though my mother expressed unrelenting concern, virtually everyone in the gym along with my P.E. teachers and classmates spurted unbridled approval. "You look amazing," they'd say to me. "How did you get so thin? Wow, you're so dedicated. I wish I could be like you."

No one had ever told me he or she wished to be like me. (Or, if someone had, I'd tuned it out and opted to focus on the onslaught of "you're stupid" and "shut up" my peers had spat at me for years.) Few people had lauded my appearance prior to my embrace of fitness. Here was a realm in which I could be somebody, even if I feared continually and often lost sleep over the prospect that if I took any time off—if I reneged on my daily rituals of lifting, burning, stretching, counting calories—it would all fall apart. (Like the Twin Towers or my parents' marriage.) Fitness, the gym, and exercise, I convinced myself, were things I could hold on to. Glue myself to. Be rendered acceptable through. Love without fearing abandonment.

Fitness would become my identity as high school went on. I'd grapple on and off with anorexia and binge eating throughout college. I took a semester off after my freshman year to log a few months at an inpatient eating disorder clinic where I was told that my issues with food were much easier to treat than my issues with exercise. No sooner had I signed myself out after my weight reached a healthier number than I was back at the gym, cycling through obsessive routines all over again, fueled in large part by a recent breakup with a long-distance boyfriend. I gripped these gym regimens like a security blanket to cover my heartbreak as well as to insulate me from the uncertainties of transferring to another college, which I was also in the process of doing.

Unlike my issues with eating, no one expressed concern about my exercise habits. That I would go to the gym two or more hours a day, that I would cancel plans with friends to take on extra workouts, that I would sneak out of movies to do jump squats and push-ups in public bathrooms was deemed *outstanding* or *inspiring* to nearly everyone who knew me. Amid the cultural hysteria over the ills of sedentarism in response to a so-called obesity epidemic, awareness of upper limits to physical activity (and its potential excess) is (no pun intended) slim. Calls for moderation in movement, the importance of off days, and the social, emotional, and physical consequences of too much time spent in motion are crowded out by our American obsession with burning fat, pursuing thinness, and trying to look like the men and women we see on the covers of fitness magazines or ads for weight loss supplements.

Who could blame my friends for not noticing I had a severe problem? The results of my tireless consumption of fitness advice and arduous workout schedules were socially laudable. Rather than putting on weight, developing jaundice, making track marks on my arms, or spending days in bed recovering from hangovers, as one suffering from other addictions might experience, I was muscular, energetic, svelte, and full of physical stamina (at least during what I'd later view as the initial stages of my lifelong struggle).

As the years went on, I inevitably developed those aches and pains brought about by refusing to rest and pushing through discomfort. Every morning I'd do an hour of yoga with the conviction that it was *healthy* no matter how hard I pushed myself. This led to a bulging disc in my lower back. Did I relent? Absolutely not. I pulled and twisted and arched my spine in the morning without warming up, only to hit the pavement after classes or my twice-weekly internship for hour-long runs. Soon enough, I was diagnosed with a severe herniation in my lumbar vertebrae after an MRI revealed a cringeworthy protrusion several vertebrae above my sacrum.

Against doctor's orders, I stuck to my rigorous, daily workouts of two hours (or more) a day. The vast majority of that time was spent hunched over an elliptical machine, pursing my lips and wincing through pain. I refused to have surgery, as was clinically recommended, because it would mean too much time off from the gym.

I'd planned to become a personal trainer after graduating college, despite what professors had told me were my academic strengths in writing and psychology. Better to be in a gym, I figured, where I'd have constant access to fitness equipment (not to mention a free health club membership) than be chained to a desk all day, unable to burn enough calories or build enough muscle to feel *okay* in my skin.

My terror of stillness pervaded every aspect of my daily life. Most noticeably, the significance of any relationship I had was punctured by my prioritization of the gym—herniated disc (and all occasional illnesses) notwithstanding. (One boyfriend literally pulled me off an elliptical machine screaming to the gym staff that I'd had a fever of 100 degrees earlier that morning. Another told me I was "sick," remarking that my painstaking pursuit of fitness was "gross" and "disturbing.") I canceled numerous plans with friends, avoided vacations, and shied away from applying to many jobs for fear that their accompanying obligations would prevent me from being "active enough."

Although I'd rail against moderation, however, I secretly craved a reason to slow down and ease off. I wanted to taper down, I wanted to enjoy life, but I didn't feel that I could—I didn't believe I was worthy of it. In my head, burning a *minimum* of 450 calories a day; lifting, lunging, and squatting on most days of the week; and performing push-ups, pull-ups, handstands, backbends, and other core-engaging arm balances were a means of protecting myself against my "natural" state—one I associated with unacceptability and worthlessness. I knew that taking time off would be "objectively" good for me—I'd read all you could read on the benefits of rest for building strength and endurance, and I was aware of the consequences too much cardio has on your heart. But I didn't trust what would happen if I altered my workouts in any significant way. I felt out of control. Unquenchable. While I ached for a sign that I was alright, acceptable, and deserving of love in the absence of my routines, I was virtually incapable of believing any evidence that would have confirmed this.

Eventually, the disc herniation got so bad that I *had* to do other things besides the gym, if only to distract myself from the physical suffering and emotional angst of unyielding pain. Not having a job straight out of college, I had far too much time on my hands, which only amplified the shaky sense of identity loss and lack of purpose resulting from having to rein in my fitness pursuits due to an injury.

I needed something significant enough to unhinge my obsessive focus from my own body, from how much it could do in a given day, and from how worthless it was if it didn't accomplish this many reps, that many circuits, or some unnecessarily lengthy number of minutes jogging or cycling. And so I began volunteering on a suicide prevention hotline in Manhattan. (A logical jump, one could argue, for someone prone to extremes like myself.)

In addition to finding an incredibly helpful therapist and committing to weekly sessions that forced me to alter my gym schedule, an enormous force in my emergence from exercise addiction began with this hotline. Hearing the stories of hundreds of people whose suffering equaled or surpassed my own made me feel less alone in the world. Moreover, "being there" for anonymous callers from all walks of life made me feel that I had some value other than how fit or in shape I appeared. On the hotline, my body was peripheral to my listening skills, my ability to remain calm under stress, and my commitment to being present for others. Here was a meaningful endeavor that rendered sitting still not so awful, an experience that lifted me out of the self-destructive abyss of solitary gym sessions that perpetuated self-hatred and eroded my energy levels, vitality, and interest in the rest of the world.

The more plugged in I became to life outside of the gym, the better I felt—even if this particular volunteer post entailed a fair amount of its own on-the-job stress. I began making more plans with friends, spending downtime with family, and even getting back on the dating circuit. I began seeing a therapist with whom I could openly discuss my obsessive focus on physical activity and the ways I'd let it get in the way of the rest of my life. More importantly, I started looking at what exactly the "rest of my life" entailed—everything from movie and music preferences to hobbies and career goals. Not surprisingly, my workouts became far more manageable during this time, enabling me to discover that existence could actually be fun again. Flexible. Free.

I began taking improvisational comedy classes, if not to balance the seriousness of my volunteer work, then to try something new. Increasingly, I found myself more open to new experiences. After a much-needed and memorable vacation with my father to New Mexico, I returned to my Manhattan home to a surprise job offer from the magazine I'd interned at during my senior year in college. Suddenly, I realized, I was feeling like a human being—validated, valuable, and worthy of rest, care, and love irrespective of how many calories I burned or how much weight I could lift.

I still went to the gym in the mornings, before my 9:00 to 6:00 pm office hours. But my workouts were restricted by the necessity of needing energy to think, to problem solve, and to be present on the job. Here was another source of self-esteem unrelated to my fitness prowess, one that equaled the satisfaction I used to feel. Moreover, I was a part of something greater than myself and my gym routines. I was a seemingly necessary component of an editorial team, on the masthead of a publication I'd wanted to work at for years, accountable for basic duties, deadlines, and assignments whose importance eclipsed my ruminations about body weight and size.

The best part? My back pain slowly started to ease as I altered my workouts. And what was once my greatest fear—that my body would significantly alter in size, shape, and acceptability if my workout routines changed in the slightest—proved to be entirely unfounded. If anything, I felt even better in my skin, realizing that my self-worth was not wholly dependent on my body fat percentage.

That's not to say that I haven't since slipped back into overzealous exercise schedules from time to time. In truth, when times got tough at that job—and the next ones I'd have down the line—I'd dip out of meetings early and sneak out on lunch breaks for a second gym session, obsess over the muscularity of my arms and torso, or find my mind latching onto the fear of not having enough time to run or do yoga.

For a time, vacations weren't the easiest, either. In the absence of a routine I tend to feel shaky. I find comfort in having access to a gym when I travel, if not only to knock out a quick workout session before or after sightseeing but that so I can let go of the worry that I'm not *doing enough* on a leisure trip. That said, I've found trips incredibly useful in rehearsing my familiarity with flexibility—which sometimes means (brace yourself) *no gym*. Traveling, especially with my fiancé (whom I can talk to openly about my anxiety and who has helped show me how to approach working out in a more feasible manner), is critical to forcing me out of the rigid thought patterns I default to, which all too easily encapsulate me in an obsessive cycle.

I've learned that I need to set up my environment so that I'm obligated to engage with other people and embrace new activities. Going to new places, committing to plans with family and friends, and challenging myself with new experiences are all part of living a healthier lifestyle. Sometimes I feel the effort it takes to keep myself from slipping into a compulsive habit of exercising equals the effort many folks need to get to the gym in the first place. (I often joke with my friends that I was born with a superpower to make the healthiest behaviors magically turn pathological.)

No matter how many hiccups I've had, however, I do know now, on a deeply ingrained level, that there is far more to my life than the gym—even if I still consider fitness a huge part of my life. My relationship to myself, my exercise behavior, and my body image aren't always perfectly sound. I'm not sure they ever will be. I default to self-destruction as a coping mechanism, especially as it involves controlling my physical appearance, and I have to work hard to not take the easier route I've grown so accustomed to involving self-harm. But unlike in college or shortly thereafter, today I'm far more attuned to my body's signals. Injury taught me this. As did practice in reorienting my focus away from how much I hated myself to what good I could do in the world.

I know now when to ease off during a workout, when to go "lighter" at the gym or to take a few days off from heavy lifting and hard cardio. I've also learned to sniff out the warning signals that what I'm doing at the gym might not be in my best interest. If I'm feeling isolated in my workouts, if I'm consistently angry, grumpy, or easily irritated after several exercise sessions in a row, I know I need to change something.

Some days, this means simply making a point to spend quality time with my fiancé or scheduling a night out with one of my close friends. Other days, I know I need to make my workout secondary to a particular task at hand—say, an assignment that's due, a deadline, or an important meeting I need to put first.

Other red flags include repeating the same exercise over a number of days and feeling compelled to perform a specific routine prior to accomplishing anything else in my day. I know when I pick up on these patterns to reach out to my therapist, to talk with my fiancé, or to force myself to switch up my exercise routine either by taking a time-limited fitness class, scheduling a meeting during the time I'd normally spend alone on a cardio machine, or going outside for a walk rather than checking in at my local sports club.

I don't believe I'll ever not want to work out. I'm an active person by nature and I need a physical outlet to channel my energy levels. I see nothing wrong with deriving self-esteem from fitness, nor do I see the gym as an inherently unhealthy way to de-stress or induce more focus.

For me, exercise crosses the line from healthy to harmful when it becomes a means of insulating myself from other people, punishing myself, and perpetually avoiding the inevitable human reality of feeling vulnerable. My exercise routines become problematic when I cling to them so as to avoid my deep fears of abandonment, my internalized sense of inferiority, and my desire to feel in total (some might say delusional) control of my appearance.

It's astonishing to me how simple it is to pull myself out of my neurosis, yet how insurmountable it sometimes seems to me before I make the effort to do so. One huge motivator that helps keep me going, however, is knowing that I am not alone in this. Sharing my story, reaching out to others, and spreading knowledge about exercise addiction has helped me find additional purpose in life apart from constant physical movement.

Of course, my story is just one of many. And while it may be unique, there are many paths into (and out of) exercise addiction. I encourage you to continue reading for more insight into others' journeys.

KAILA PRINS

Kaila, a California-based marketing copywriter and health coach, also traces the roots of her battles with exercise addiction to childhood. "The whole thing started when I was thirteen—I was this average, slightly chubby kid," Kaila recalls. "I got a gym membership so I had something to do after summer camp and I had no idea what I was doing."

What began as a healthy pastime soon turned into an obsession. No sooner had Kaila discovered the euphoria brought about by her thirty-minute Stairmaster sessions than she set out to push her physical limits as far as she could. "I'd do dance warm-ups, sit-ups, butterfly kicks, donkey kicks—all these stupid things in my room before bedtime. I'd go to the gym every day before school, staying longer each time and biking three miles there and back." By the end of junior high, at five feet, four inches tall, Kaila weighed a meager ninety-seven pounds.

After a serious setback involving a bone tumor in her knee resolved only by surgery in ninth grade, Kaila promised herself she'd bounce back into working out. She joined her high school's cross country team and committed to becoming a runner.

Like most athletes, Kaila rejoiced in the competition her sport entailed. Especially when she bested her male friends in speed, distance, or frequency. By the end of high school Kaila was racing twice a day.

Cut to college, where Kaila's pursuit of fitness was curtailed to a more moderate level by the demands of a rigorous academic schedule. Kaila was deeply involved in the theater community at the New York City–based institution where she spent her freshman year, and she carried this passionate interest with her when she transferred to a college in her home state of Florida to finish her degree.

With the weather change came a wardrobe change, and Kaila soon found herself among bikini-clad girls sporting bodies she considered more toned and fit than hers. Less challenged by her new college environment and hyper-aware of what she perceived as her personal flaws, Kaila forced herself back into a daily running regimen.

Getting nothing but praise from her peers, she kept going. Not only did she increase the time she spent hitting the pavement, but she slashed her caloric intake as much as possible, biked several miles to the nearest gym on a daily basis, added an additional fifty minutes of stair climbing to her routine of pull-ups, push-ups, and free weights, and often threw in an additional afternoon tennis match with a pal.

When Kaila landed a summer study abroad opportunity in England that promised her no gym access, she invested in a weighted jump rope to use every night—with a minimum workout time of twenty minutes, she told herself—and ran through the blustery Cambridge weather day in and day out.

Kaila went on to run the theater department at a high school in Boca Raton, Florida, after graduating from college. After a stressful year spent teaching more than two hundred students while directing three plays, designing curricula for five classes, and running two clubs, Kaila crossed paths with a man whose obsession with fitness equaled her own. Her relationship with exercise became even more engulfing as the two began dating and, eventually, living together. Infatuated with the size of his muscles—and the diet that made them pop—his 4:00 am wake-up call to hit the gym before normal business hours rubbed off on Kaila. Not only did he introduce her to the squats and dead lifts by which she'd later be injured, but he also expounded on the virtues of female fitness models' physiques. Acutely attuned to the pressure to look good, to build more muscle, and to be as thin and fit as she possibly could,

Kaila quickly absorbed her boyfriend's perspective—pushing herself so hard over the course of two weeks that she developed a painfully severe case of plantar fasciitis.

Sleep became an impediment to Kaila's goals at the gym and she refused to relent in her tireless pursuit of physical perfection. "I was religious about working out," she recalls of the months she attempted to pummel her body into the shapes she saw on magazine covers. "My entire life was contingent upon whether I could get to the gym in the morning." The gym was at once her sole coping mechanism as well as a prime cause of her mood imbalances and social withdrawal—not to mention a host of physical ailments ranging from menstrual irregularities to torn ligaments and bone swelling. "The only time I ever felt good was when I was exercising," Kaila says. "I was dependent on exercise in order to function."

A few months into graduate school, Kaila's sense of entrapment burgeoned. Her irritability peaked, her interest in sex was virtually null, she was angry, depressed, and she toiled to keep thoughts of suicide out of her mind. "I knew I needed help," Kaila admits. "I'd given up my dreams of getting a PhD in exchange for an International Federation of Bodybuilding card."

Hoping to finance a recovery program, Kaila found a job working in retail. Where others may have found stress in the long hours (and customer management skills) the gig often entailed, Kaila discovered a surprising refuge from her relentless gym schedule. "I just couldn't keep it up anymore," she says. "I worked about sixty hours a week and I ended up loving it. I still went to the gym in the morning but sometimes I worked until eleven at night so I couldn't always get up that early." Slowly but surely, the structure of her new job enabled Kaila to emerge from a self-destructive rut and reorient her mind toward tasks unrelated to how muscular or thin she could render her body. "Honestly, I feel like that job saved my life," Kaila says. "I had a chance to focus on other people. I ended up putting on a little bit of weight but I was okay with that."

Going forward, it wasn't all uphill—after injuring her ankle during a run, undergoing several ankle surgeries, and receiving a tentative diagnosis of complex regional pain syndrome—and Kaila was able to find other means of relating to the world apart from superhuman amounts of activity. Physically incapable of pushing herself to the extremes she'd formerly suffered through, Kaila occupied her off time from work beginning a blog, founding a podcast, and studying to get certified as a health coach. She's since left retail (and Florida) to work at a marketing company in California during the day and she loves the new challenges its nine-to-five tasks pose to her brain. When she's not immersed in all the above, Kaila's probably out walking her Chihuahua or curling up on the couch to watch Nickelodeon with her younger brother. (After a brief respite from work due to disability, Kaila relocated to her family's new home in California.)

When she thinks about the days she spent destroying her body for the supposed sake of fitness, she shudders. "My whole goal was not to be human. I remember losing my period for the first time and feeling like it was the best day ever because I was that much closer to not being a real woman." Though Kaila still battles the critical voice in her head that fueled her addictive exercise habits, she's learned to unlatch her attention from honing her fitness regimens to helping others—and to taking daily moments to reflect on what she's grateful for.

No longer chasing the humanless form of a mannequin, Kaila's gradually grown more comfortable in her skin. "I don't have a yoga body and I wasn't meant to look like a fitness model," she says. "I'm a mesomorph—I retain fat on my hips and I have an hourglass figure. I just have to deal. But I'm normal now. I've got breasts again and love handles. I'm okay with that."

Since giving up her arduous workout schedule—in large part a consequence of the injuries she incurred after pushing herself too hard for too long—Kaila's also gained a much wiser perspective. "The silver lining in my journey is that I'm actually thankful for all the awful experiences I've had. They've made me a better, stronger, and more aware person." Whether you're struggling with an eating disorder, an alcohol or drug problem, or an addiction to exercise, Kaila says, "when you get to the other side—when you're forced to recover through intervention by other people or by your body giving up—you become more empathetic, sensitive, and less obsessed with yourself."

A large part of Kaila's newfound awareness entails some serious media literacy—reading through the messages fitness magazines use to promote supplements, weight loss regimens, or simply to sell copy, as well as taking the time to connect with family, friends, and coworkers. "I actually go out and have fun now," Kaila says. "I'm able to do things I never could have done before because I was so fixated on getting up at 4:00 am to time my oatmeal before the gym."

Things are certainly looking up for Kaila these days, but she hasn't come out of her exercise addiction unscathed. Her menstrual cycle still hasn't returned and she's recently undergone yet another surgery to fix the ankle injury incurred during her former days of fitness overdrive.

"I'm twenty-seven years old and I haven't had a period in almost two years," Kaila says. "I just want to be a normal functioning woman again. I never saw myself as someone to get married and have kids, but now that I might not be able to, it's the scariest, most awful thing ever. Part of why I'm motivated to be a health coach is to help other women avoid doing to themselves what I did to myself through exercise—and potentially destroying a big part of their future."

C

C grew up in a household where the importance of fitness was heavily stressed and a regular exercise regimen was strongly encouraged. Cognizant of her comparatively taller size and struggling with low self-esteem throughout middle school, C delighted in the changes brought about to her body by running on her high school track team.

Running granted C a sense of empowerment—a refuge from the self-consciousness of hitting puberty well before the rest of the girls in her fifth grade class and an escape from the voices of peers who called her "Amazon" and "bowling ball" due to her tall height. Wanting more relief, C convinced her parents to let her join a gym close to her school and began running four to five miles each day on the treadmill before classes—even on days she had track practice.

This doubled physical activity still didn't satisfy C. In response to a nagging sense that she had to *do more*, she increased her physical activity levels further. Whereas she'd previously woken at 5:30 to run before school, she now felt the need to lace up her running shoes at 4:00 am, just to get in *enough*.

C lost an unhealthy amount of weight. She also began obsessing over her dwindling size. Soon she began vomiting after meals, consuming diet pills, and taking laxatives. No matter how depleted she became, however, C persisted in hitting the pavement day in and day out.

"I ran whenever I ate any of the foods on my 'bad list,'" says C. "I ran when I was sad. I ran when I was angry. I ran until I fainted. I ran in thunderstorms and hurricanes. I ran with fevers and kidney infections. I ran until my body began to fight back. My toenails cracked and fell off. My knees and ankles began to ache horribly and would keep me up at night. I began to run with ankle braces and knee braces on each leg, ignoring the confused looks of bystanders as I limped past them."

Deprived and exhausted, C's compulsive thought patterns raced out of control. Her menstrual cycle ceased, she battled severe insomnia, she experienced constant physical pain, and she began losing her hair. Emotionally, she cycled between depression and numbness. "I started disassociating during random moments—in class, with my family, even when I was driving," C remembers. "I would suddenly feel dizzy and confused, very far away from whatever was in front of me. I worried that I wasn't real anymore."

C's identity and self-worth were so enmeshed in how many miles she logged and how thin she appeared that she lost hold on who she was apart from exercise. "I prided myself on self-discipline. I was afraid if I missed a workout, I would become like everyone else. Losing my self-discipline would mean that I had nothing left that made me special—nothing to be proud of." She even delighted in the "personal whipping routine" that her pain-filled runs granted her. She felt they were required in order for her to justify basic comforts and amenities, such as something as simple as a post-workout shower. "The pain made me feel like I was actually doing something—correcting how lazy, sloppy, and stupid I felt I was," C says. Without her unsustainably arduous running schedule, C admits, she feared no one would care about her.

Running wasn't the only way C punished herself. Throughout high school and her first two years of college, she cut her arms and thighs. Shame and guilt hung over her head constantly. "I felt like I was the wet blanket among my friends, the uptight one who couldn't let loose. Even though this is essentially what I had always wanted, it did not feel good."

Like most exercise addicts, C withdrew from the majority of social activities available to her, declining invitations to dinners or evening events for fear that staying out too late might throw off her morning routine. She was continuously tired and barely able to focus. As a consequence of her self-destruction, her academic performance began suffering almost as much as her health. Perpetually on edge due to her ever-increasing hunger for exercise and her avoidance of pleasure, C fought regularly with her friends, parents, and her significant other.

Despite her family's repeated attempts to draw attention to the severity of her compulsive exercise and restrictive eating habits, C strenuously resisted help. Torn between wanting to be recognized for her efforts and being angered when those close to her encouraged her to seek help, C was aware that she had a problem yet remained unwilling to change. While C cannot peg one specific moment as the turning point that prompted her to seek treatment, she does recall a series of cumulative events that gradually opened her eyes to how engulfed she'd become in her overzealous exercise habits.

C remembers seeing a book about eating disorders on her father's nightstand, a silent admission that he was truly concerned and not just trying to control her (as she'd previously assumed). She also remembers a conversation she had with a therapist she'd been seeing regarding the consequences of losing her period. C wanted to have children at some point in her life but realized she would compromise this goal by remaining too thin. "Eventually," C says, "I just realized either I was going to die or I could give this another shot."

Thankfully, C chose the latter.

She enrolled herself in an intensive outpatient program geared toward addressing body image and eating disturbances, worked with a nutritionist to get her weight back to a functional level, continued seeing an individual therapist, and attended group therapy.

Eager not to lose steam on her work toward an undergraduate degree, C persevered through college courses throughout her treatment—a decision she later came to regret. "Sometimes I do wish I'd just gone inpatient," C admits. "I feel like I lost years of progress due to my stubbornness in not going." Nevertheless, C stuck with her commitment to getting better. Despite some setbacks at the beginning of graduate school—without a therapist or dietician, C began running twice daily and dropping weight again while averaging four hours of sleep on most nights—she linked up with a new dietician and therapist to help get her back on track. Four years later, C still sees the same therapist, who has helped her hone coping mechanisms like positive self-talk and behavioral change.

One of C's biggest challenges has been resisting the urge to run every morning at 5:00 am. "Initially, it was mentally excruciating to stay in bed in the morning. I had to literally talk to myself out loud, reiterating that it was okay to sleep and to respect my body."

It took about six months, C remembers, before she stopped feeling guilty and anxious for taking weekends off to recover. "It was like an internal war all the time inside of myself," she says. "I felt horrible guilt for not running or even just for waiting to run."

Slowly but surely, C emerged from her obsessive thoughts, freeing her mind and her time up for other pursuits—like the doctorate degree in clinical psychology she's finishing up. (Her specialization? Eating disorders.)

C never wrote off exercise entirely. She continues to run about four miles several times each week. Though she still admits feeling "a bit over-regimented and rigid about exercise," she's able to successfully cut herself off when she hears that compulsive voice in her head urging her to push past her limits. "I'm better able now to talk myself out of the guilt or anxiety I feel if I miss a day or don't do 'enough.'"

Silencing the echoes of a disordered mind-set still takes effort. "I have to constantly work to differentiate whether my eating disorder is doing the talking or whether the thoughts I'm having about my body and behavior are coming from me," says C. But a strong marker of her admirable progress is the shift in her assumption that she *must* workout despite illness and injury: "If I need to sleep in the morning, I do. If I feel sick, I stay home. I know how to listen to my body now."

C has also worked hard with her therapist to find coping skills other than running. These days, when she's feeling frustrated, lonely, sad, or angry, she's more likely to reach out to a friend or family, bake, write, or read. She also enjoys playing board games with her fiancé and planning movie nights with close friends.

Locating the self underneath her compulsive exercise habits continues to be a struggle for C—albeit a more manageable one as each day in her recovery goes by. "I don't believe it's completely gone or will ever be," C says. "But I know I can't go back to where I was again, because I don't want to lose what I have in my life now."

C recognizes the challenges of overcoming an addiction to exercise, as well as an eating disorder. Unlike kicking a habit with substance abuse, "you can't walk away from exercise or food—you *have* to practice moderation. You don't have a choice to be abstinent."

It's taken her years but C takes heart in the assurance that "people love me. And I love me—for me. Not because I'm thin and I exercise a lot." In the event she begins to doubt this, C has learned to stop herself and ask, "What do I really want to be remembered for? Being skinny and fit? Or accomplishing something meaningful in my lifetime?"

CHARLOTTE ANDERSEN

For Charlotte, gymnastics was the one constant in a life spent moving around the country following her dad's job as a contractor with the Air Force. Handstands, flips, flying, and other callisthenic feats kept her and her siblings entertained when making new friends felt increasingly pointless. Even though she recalls being a mediocre gymnast at best, she loved the sport so much that she felt a great desire to get better and please her coaches. This led her to seek out any way possible to excel, including manipulating her body. "Being a gymnast really shaped a lot of my views on exercise and fitness," Charlotte says, "the lighter you were, the higher you flew—there was a lot of emphasis placed on keeping our weight down."

Charlotte believes her relationship with physical activity remained relatively healthy for the majority of her childhood and adolescence. Her eating habits, however, did not. Fighting a perfectionist streak and hoping to manipulate her tall form into the smaller size preferred by her coaches, Charlotte started restricting her food in middle school. Counting calories and fat grams made her feel in control of a life over whose trajectory she felt she had a negligible influence. By the time she was in college she was using vegetarianism as a justification for her painfully rigid diet.

Maintaining her austere diet when surrounded by typical college foods like pizza and chips became increasingly difficult and she found herself bingeing on "safe foods." But one day she panicked that she'd eaten too much and tried to make herself purge. After spending hours gagging over the toilet to no avail, she realized what a terrible situation she was in and telephoned her parents for help. She also got in touch with an outpatient therapist and enrolled in campus support groups to keep herself afloat. Nine months later, she felt she was back on track as far as her eating disorder was concerned. But the specter of self-destruction would shadow her behaviors once again following the birth of her third child, years after graduation.

Charlotte met her husband during graduate school. He, too, was studying for a degree in computer information systems. Diplomas in hand, the couple conceived their first child in 2001. They were devastated when Charlotte gave birth to a baby girl who was stillborn due to complications of Turner's syndrome, a genetic disorder. Even though the doctors assured her that her daughter's death was in no way her fault, Charlotte privately wondered if the years of abuse she'd put her body through were to blame. "This grief is the kind that reminds me I have a smoldering coal of hurt deep inside," Charlotte poignantly writes of the traumatic experience on her blog, *The Great Fitness Experiment*, "one that still burns tears into my eyes." Though the lurch back into normal life was physically and psychologically arduous, Charlotte and her husband eventually held out hope long enough to bring a second child into the world, followed by three more.

But just because Charlotte's approach to nutrition was sound enough to render her body capable of normal functioning didn't mean she was invulnerable to triggers that risked sending her back down a path of self-destruction. Just before her second son was born she got a disturbing unexpected call from a detective. The police had recently arrested a man for multiple counts of sexual assault. Charlotte knew him all too well. She had dated him, briefly, in college, and was one of his first victims.

Although with the help of Charlotte's testimony justice was eventually served—the perpetrator was sentenced to prison the day before her second son was born—participating in the case kicked off a wave of traumatic memories that made Charlotte desperate to escape. Clinging to the goal of shedding postpartum pounds, Charlotte promised herself she'd focus on getting her body back in shape so as to distract herself from unbearably painful emotions.

Her first exercise of choice became running. "It was the easiest to do around my kids' schedules," Charlotte explains. "I'd run so hard and so fast that I couldn't think about anything but my legs pounding against the pavement. It was a means of dissociating from painful feelings that I didn't know what to do with. I felt so dirty and unclean and I worried that people would see that. I thought if I could make my body perfect, if I could be skinny, people wouldn't see what a mess I was. I thought I could heal myself from the outside in." Charlotte also delighted in the unmatched rush of endorphins that physical activity naturally afforded her, rescuing her from the waves of anxiety and panic attacks she'd been cycling through since revisiting her earlier trauma.

Running was soon amplified by kickboxing, followed by aerobics, weight lifting, dance classes, and the use of numerous cardiovascular machines (ellipticals, Stairmasters, you name it). Charlotte began *The Great Fitness Experiment* to catalog her seemingly healthy attempts to try every possible fitness craze out there. Quickly gaining followers, she ultimately landed a book deal from her astounding documentation of it all.

Awash in praise from readers who applauded Charlotte's above-average exercise habits, she didn't realize how the blog was rekindling a disordered relationship with her body. "I thought I was being super healthy," Charlotte admits. "I would tell people that I used to be anorexic but I was recovered now and that I was so glad I found fitness. I feel bad now about the responsibility I had to my readers."

Charlotte's ostensibly "healthy" pursuits came to a crisis point when she was training for a marathon. Accustomed to working out for up to six hours a day—once in the morning after dropping the kids off at school, once in the afternoon, and again at night after putting the kids to sleep—Charlotte returned from a twenty-six-mile run dehydrated and famished. But rather than refueling and letting herself recover, Charlotte couldn't wrap her mind around missing her regular kickboxing class. On no food or fluid, Charlotte completed the class. By then, her heart was beating erratically and she felt like she was going to throw up. She ran into the hallway to find a garbage can and promptly fainted. A friend carried her downstairs, past the day-care room where her kids watched with horror as she lay on the floor shaking and crying.

This was exactly what Charlotte's husband was afraid of. He had suspected for a while that her behavior had gotten out of control, not to mention feeling neglected by her absence as she spent more time sweating than connecting with him. The day she fainted, he'd even tried to stop her from going to the gym by hiding her running shoes and taking her car keys. (Charlotte circumvented his intervention by locating an old pair of sneakers and a spare set of keys.)

When Charlotte came to, heart still palpitating and head spinning, she finally saw how bad her exercise addiction had become. "I didn't want my kids to see me like that ever again," she recalls. "I knew in that moment that I needed to get help. I knew I needed to take care of their mother and I was suddenly scared."

Knowing that she needed someone to keep her accountable for her own health, Charlotte reached out to several eating disorder professionals in her area. She ended up sticking with a once-weekly appointment with her therapist, committing to group work, and seeing a nutritionist to help recalibrate her weight in the wake of a dangerously low body fat percentage resulting from too much time spent burning it all off. Charlotte was also incredibly open about her struggles on her blog. She came clean about her struggles, pinpointing the all-too-easily hidden realities of exercise addiction and invited her readers to call her out should any of her future posts hint of renewed excess. Charlotte's readers ended up being immensely supportive of her recovery process. Many of them, in fact, even came out with their own struggles related to exercise addiction and body image disorders.

Charlotte's path back to proper health wasn't without setbacks. She was dealt a huge blow when her doctor determined her previous over-exertion had led to her development of hypothyroidism. This caused her to put on weight, to lose her hair, to stop menstruating, and destabilized her electrolytes, making her continually feel cold and depressed. In addition, she had stress fractures in her shins and feet. To allow her body to heal from years of overtraining, Charlotte was prescribed a complete eight-week rest from all exercise.

Transitioning from spending the majority of her days in motion to avoiding strenuous physical activity at all costs was devastating to Charlotte, who not only kissed good-bye that exercise-induced endorphin rush during the time it took her to get back on track, but also parted ways with her social group. A large part of Charlotte's recovery involved the difficult step of disconnecting with her previous fitness pals. Much like a recovering alcoholic or addict who must remove him- or herself from tempting influences so as to prevent relapse, many exercise addicts find it helpful to nurture relationships with less exercise-obsessed friends. "Hearing my old friends from the gym talk about exercise all the time was so hard for me," Charlotte recalls. "They would tell me, 'Oh, you don't have a problem. We exercise just as much as you do and we're okay.' That was really triggering. Sometimes I'd cry after they left."

Of the first weeks spent back in reality, Charlotte recalls feeling as if she'd lost everything she knew. It took her two months before her body resumed its balance. And after it did, she carefully monitored her resumption of exercise, following her therapist and doctor's guidelines to exercise no more than one hour a day with a cap of five days per week.

Echoing the sentiments of many former exercise addicts, Charlotte agrees that the phrase "exercise in moderation" means little, if anything, to her obsession-prone brain. "I need to hear a number. I still need to have limits," Charlotte says.

Charlotte also required additional outlets to manage her anxiety and combat boredom that didn't involve overdoing it at the gym. In addition to therapy and a pharmaceutical regimen of daily antidepressants, Charlotte devoted even more time to playing with her kids, writing her blog and books, volunteering at the church she attends with her family, reading, and crocheting. Breath work and yoga have become invaluable tools in her new self-survival kit, and she credits meditation for enabling her to learn how to navigate panic attacks rather than (literally) running away from them.

With the help of a strong team of mental and physical health professionals along with the unflagging support of her husband, Charlotte was able to get back on track. Today, she limits herself to five days a week of exercise, keeping the total time spent per session to one hour, tops. She keeps herself in check by continuing to write about her fitness habits on the Web. ("I'm still very honest about my disorder on my blog," she says. "I'll get comments from readers who think I'm doing too much again and I really pay attention. I know I don't have a good personal perspective on that—sometimes I need others to be my voice of reason.")

Charlotte can now comfortably say that her life is no longer ruled by her workout schedule. "I focus on exercises that make me feel good, not ones that are punishing," she says with a newfound calmness. This means that on some days exercise boils down to leisurely walks with friends around her neighborhood or a stress-reducing series of yoga postures alone in her room. "I can recognize now when my body needs a rest and I grant it that. I don't count calories and I no longer keep an obsessive tab on my heart rate," Charlotte explains. Nor, she adds, does she feel the need to "earn" her food or punish herself for eating something "bad" by exercising.

Charlotte continues to meet with her therapist when she needs an emotional tune-up (or check-in). And she's proud to proclaim that she and her husband are stronger than ever. "I finally have time to relax," Charlotte says. In between writing, interviewing people for articles she pens as a freelancer, and raising four children, Charlotte derives immense gratification from finding ways to help others. The happiness she's been able to find in interpersonal connection, she believes, far outweighs any high you could ever get from hitting the gym.

B

B's first introduction to exercise was a volunteer challenge sponsored by Nike. Participants were given individual pedometers and competed to log as many kilometers as possible over a several week span. B delighted in how good running made her feel, along with the relief it afforded her from the stresses of settling into a new school and making new friends. She'd just begun high school in a town her family had recently moved to following her father's relocation for work. B recalls how her exercise habits quickly started blooming: "Each run grew slightly longer, and when I finished the challenge, I kept running," she recalls. B had also gotten involved with her school's rowing team, which reinforced her attempts to keep fit, especially over holidays. No sooner had her running grown in rigor and intensity than she began feeling "it was a habit that I could not get through the day without." B's weight dropped— she'd started eating less under the assumption it would to make running easier—but despite medical advice to tone down her cardiovascular output she kept increasing her distance, striving toward what she saw as perfection.

"These runs became part of my daily schedule," B says, "something I had to do to get through the day. It became ingrained in my head that if I hadn't been for a run, somehow I couldn't function properly." B would get moody without reason, lash out at her parents and two sisters, and cycle through waves of depression and inexplicable sadness. She also lost her appetite. Though she briefly regained weight with the help of a dietician in about six weeks, she found herself slipping back into an even more obsessive focus on exercise during her senior year. "I found it so hard to sit down and study for long periods of time without knowing in my mind that I had exercised," says B. Some days B would feel the need to run three times a day, in addition to performing strength and conditioning exercises, just to be able to sit still.

B believes her exercise addiction hit its lowest point after she happened upon cycling. No sooner had she mastered riding a bike than it topped her list of daily obligatory routines. She'd run in the morning, bike for an hour in the afternoon, and continue to strength train throughout.

Eventually, B's habits led to injuries so severe she could no longer run. Her iliotibial bands became so stiff that she could barely walk and her knees started locking. Instead of scaling back to let her body heal, B increased her workouts, swimming for hours a day, "cycling like crazy," and spending even more time conditioning. As soon as the pain of her injuries became manageable, she went right back to running.

Due to B's subsequent weight loss from added activities, yet another dietician advised her to put exercise on hold until she achieved a healthier body mass index. But B told the dietician point-blank that this was impossible, persuading her instead to green-light one twenty-minute bike ride per day. "Little did anyone know," B says, "that I was doing exercises in the morning before breakfast and running up and down the stairs in our house whenever I was alone." She'd also sneak in runs during her high school's free periods, secreting herself away from friends to perform intervals of sprinting and speed-walking outside. Exercise offered B a relief from her worries, an ability to relax, and a means of focusing. How could she ever entirely give it up?

Although B believes the exercise did help her offset the stress of her senior year, she admits that it markedly damaged her social life. "I would always choose exercise over anything to do with friends," she explains. Her friends noticed this, too, frequently commenting on her noticeable absence. Echoing the voices of many exercise addicts, B highlights the reason friends and family are often second to fitness: "Exercise," B says, "seems to give me more pleasure than anyone I know."

"My relationship with my older sister has also greatly suffered," B admits. "She worries about me." As do her parents. "I can't handle the way they make me feel guilty about what I'm doing," she says.

B has recently graduated from high school and continues to struggle with what she sees as a full-blown addiction. Her excessive physical activity has taken a toll on her young body. Though B is now eighteen years old, she still has never menstruated. "Most people think I'm around twelve or thirteen," she says—a visual sign of her significantly delayed puberty.

Although B has seen a sports psychologist and worked with a dietician, she finds it challenging to follow—or believe—the advice given to her. When not running, cycling, or lifting weights, B enjoys walking her dog, surfing, cooking, gardening, and "watching movies at night after I feel like I've had a good day of exercise." She and her family both hope that, with time, she may be able to let herself indulge a bit more in the pleasure these activities offer her, along with the care and attention that her family and friends want to give her.

BEN CARTER

By age seven, Ben had already experienced fitness's joys after his father, an avid exerciser, introduced him to jogging. For ten years, Ben ran just about every night until he neared the end of high school. From seventeen until twenty-two, he called it quits on his cardio regimen—"I had no need for it," Ben says. "I'd burnt myself out"—and quickly found himself slipping into a less healthy routine of drinking, smoking, and indulging in unhealthy foods.

Years later, Ben sought help from a well-meaning therapist following notable dips in his mood. To help manage his depression and anxiety, the therapist suggested Ben try giving running another go. He did. But rather than making him feel better, Ben's attempts to get back into shape made him feel even worse.

"At first I began exercising as a healthy way to escape from my symptoms," recalls Ben. He'd run every couple of days, increasing his distance and time each month. At first Ben felt relief. When compared to the years he spent on antidepressants, mood stabilizers, and antianxiety medications, exercise gave him a new, motivating focus. "It made me feel good about myself," Ben says, "proud of what I was achieving. I never had that before."

Ben likens the runner's high he experienced "to the feeling I got from drinking alcohol." The difference, however, was that Ben assumed he "could binge on it every day and the only consequence would be health and happiness." Ben went into his new embrace of fitness considering it, like many exercise addicts, "the perfect drug."

For a time, getting in shape did make Ben healthier and happier. He lost weight, built muscle, and looked forward to running and lifting. But when he eventually ran into injuries—a torn bicep, iliotibial band syndrome, sprains and strains in his ankle and knee joints—he started to suspect something was wrong.

"The routine I developed became increasingly lengthy and rigid," Ben says. " I would *have* to stick to it." As he continued to push himself past his mental and physical limits, Ben's anticipation of exercise became infused with dread. Even *during* his workouts Ben says he felt horrible. "I was in so much pain. I was dizzy and weak, and I couldn't achieve the same results as before. Sometimes I'd cry as I ran."

Yet no matter how awful Ben felt, he could not relent. "I felt like a prisoner trapped inside my head, compelled to do all these things. Exercise is the only thing that gave me that rush."

Obsession, Ben believes, is an understatement in describing his mental and physical cravings to remain in constant motion. He'd find himself "crying and shaking, just thinking about having to put my body through another session" yet unable to stop himself from hitting the pavement each day. "Exercise gave me a purpose and a meaning, something to do and to work toward. I didn't get that feeling from work, study, or social activities," he says.

As Ben's body and sanity began to crumble, so too did his social and professional life. Ben quit playing cricket—a hobby he'd enjoyed since boyhood—and lost his longtime girlfriend and even his job. He excised friends from his life who weren't active, avoided activities that entailed sitting for long stretches of time, and alienated family members—all of whom remained highly concerned, baffled, and confused by Ben's pathological relationship with a behavior that was supposed to be good for you.

"Ninety-nine percent of my mental capacity was being used to think about exercise and everything relating to it," says Ben, explaining the hold excessive physical activity had taken over his life. "If anyone got in my way of working out or if a friend or family member asked me to do them a favor when I had a run or weight training session planned I just said no. I was intolerant of anything that kept me from exercising."

The anxiety Ben felt at the prospect of missing a workout was debilitating. "If I was unable to work out or delayed from it, I would experience the classic symptoms of panic. I would be short of breath, have palpitations, and get shaky or dizzy." When not in motion, Ben's thoughts would race: "How can I get out of this situation and get my workout in?" One skipped gym session triggered a drastic plummet in his self-esteem. "I felt lazy, slothful, disgusting. I would be so disappointed in myself that I just couldn't sit with the feelings," Ben says.

The time he'd spend exercising became Ben's only relief. "After that, I'd be back to worrying about my next workout. But that hour was bliss—it was why I kept forcing myself through the pain, to get to that feeling. Exercise became the only way I could escape."

Both a psychologist and Ben's primary care physician intervened to demand he put a stop to his overzealous physical activity after Ben's weight dropped to a dangerously low level. Not only were his muscles sore and riddled with strains; they were atrophying. His joints also screamed in pain—"my body began to eat itself," Ben says. He'd even begun bingeing voraciously each night, unable to control an appetite for the proper amount of fuel to compensate for the hundreds of calories he was burning each day.

Due to the severity of his weight loss and cumulative injuries, Ben rendered himself physically incapable of running. With the help of a psychiatrist, he was able to regain enough weight to be able to walk, but he continues to feel "awful when I don't do anything—those same feelings of laziness, slothfulness, they remain." Unable to hold down a job due to the mental and physical fallout from years spent overworking his body, Ben was forced to go on disability.

He still struggles to keep physical activity within reason. "I am still very much addicted," Ben admits. "I think about exercise a lot, although nowhere nearly as much as before." Currently, Ben is working with a psychiatrist to find a workable medication regimen to manage his depression and anxiety symptoms. He continues to walk daily and he hopes to be able to return to physical activity in a non-self-destructive manner.

"I want to enjoy exercise," Ben says, "not have it consume me." Though he admits he's got a long way to go in terms of recovery, Ben is able to envision what a healthy relationship with working out would look like. "I don't think recovery is about completely avoiding exercise," he says. "It's about enjoying it within a normal range, not always being tempted to go that extra kilometer. I'd like to get there—to a point where I can take a week off without freaking out."

MYLES ALEXANDER

Triathlete Myles Alexander's relationship with physical activity wasn't always pathological. He began exercising moderately as a means to maintain muscularity, to impress his girlfriend, and to feel better in his skin during college. At the outset, his efforts were anything but harmful. They paid off handsomely. He looked and felt great, he adequately refueled after training sessions, and he maintained a successful academic and social life outside the gym. But one year into his new gym routine, an offhand remark from a woman he was dating at the time triggered an insidious seed of self-destruction to blossom in Myles's otherwise healthy attempts to be fit. "One day she told me, 'I'm just not finding you attractive anymore. Maybe you've gained a little weight,'" Myles recalls. Though he believes there were other factors predisposing him to the self-destruction that shortly ensued, he admits "that really hit me to the core. I looked in the mirror and was like, 'yeah, I could use going to the gym more.'"

Wanting to streamline his self-improvement, Myles not only increased his lifting and conditioning regimen but also cut back on his food intake. Soon he was going to the gym at least six days a week and using it as a means to purge excess calories. "If I had a hamburger I'd feel that I'd *have to* work it off," Myles recalls, pegging the onset of his exercise addiction to the moment his pursuit of fitness became obligatory rather than enjoyable. "My workouts became all about how many calories I was taking in and how many I was burning at the gym," says Myles. "It started becoming all about controlling whatever I was consuming."

Myles's focus was rapidly engulfed by an obsession with balancing what he took in and what he expended. He became fixated on the idea of constant betterment, channeling his characteristic perfectionism solely toward incinerating as much body fat as possible. "There was this switch in my head to the mind-set that *I've got to do this every day*," Myles says. "Exercise just took over my life." Trapped in an irrational mind-set, Myles "convinced myself and lied to everyone around me that what I was doing was actually good—that all this time I was spending at the gym was a reflection of how much I cared about my health." Where others saw cause for concern, Myles saw endless room for progress. Even when friends approached him to point out that he was wasting away, Myles waved their worries off under the assumption they hadn't a clue what they were talking about. "I thought I looked fantastic. Every-one around me was asking if I was sick," Myles recalls.

In addition to feeding off his ability to painstakingly pursue goals, Myles's excessive pursuit of thinness via physical activity and malnutri-tion quelled a great swell of loneliness he'd experienced after entering college, especially while studying abroad in London one year. "I felt very alone," Myles admits. "I found comfort in focusing on weight, calories, what I put in my body, and working out. The repetitive nature of it, doing the same thing every day, gave me a sense of control."

After the semester he spent abroad, even the same girlfriend who'd initially advised Myles to lose weight waved a red flag at how much time Myles was spending at the gym. Lying in bed one weekend morning next to her, Myles shot up and began getting ready to go to the gym. "I remember her asking me, 'Don't you just want to lie here?' And I was like, 'No. I just want to go to the gym.' I didn't think about it at all. I was rationalizing to myself why it was okay to shut my girlfriend down."

As Myles's anorexia and abuse of fitness continued, he eventually became too weak to walk up the stairs to his college dorm. "One day after trying to make it back to my room I just collapsed," Myles recalls. "That's really when I knew something was wrong—when I knew I was sick."

Soon after this incident, Myles arranged to see a doctor back in his hometown of Chicago. In a striking display of the pervasive ignorance surrounding eating disorders among men, not one medical professional inquired about Myles's unhealthy eating habits. "It took a while for my doctors to realize I was starving myself. I think it was because I was a guy. The *last* thing they asked about was whether I was eating enough." By that point, however, Myles's self-abuse had already taken a shocking toll. He was diagnosed with an irregular heartbeat, iron deficiency, fatty liver issues from malnutrition, early onset hair loss, swollen glands, and extreme fatigue. Bone density had also become an issue for Myles in the wake of his self-abuse, as did memory problems, depression, and difficulty achieving erection. Some of these issues took more than a year to recover from.

Despite the severity of this health scare, Myles attempted to resume his exercise habits upon returning to school after a brief medical leave—chalking his exhaustion up to a pervasive cold or potential viral infection rather than malnutrition. "That's when a coach at my school's gym took me aside and told me I needed to meet with a shrink," Myles says. Only then did he truly gain a hint of insight into how disordered his relationship with exercise and eating had become. "I was deteriorating, I needed to get healthy, and someone finally called me out on it."

Toward the end of that semester, Myles finally admitted to himself that he had a problem. He began seeing a therapist and meeting with another coach at his college who doubled as a nutritionist to review what he was eating on a daily basis. With this support, Myles was able to ratchet his weight back up to a healthier number. At this point, it was time to relearn how to exercise in a healthier manner—a careful process his coach guided him through every step of the way.

Within weeks of remastering the basics of exercise and regaining basic strength—from walking up stairs to squatting, lunging, running, and lifting—Myles put on a noticeable amount of muscle. The process wasn't easy, however. It triggered a range of former insecurities, obsessive thought patterns, and anxieties. Yet Myles's coach stood by his side, reassuring him she was there to help him get healthy, offering him a shoulder to cry on, and providing a nonjudgmental ear to which he could confess previously unspoken fears surrounding body image, identity, and self-esteem.

Through her, Myles feels he learned how to trust others again. And only with that trust could he begin to refamiliarize himself with his own body's signals (especially hunger) and feed himself lovingly. Myles believes mastering the art of knowing when to stop, take a break, or take a day off is an ongoing process, but the first steps toward greater self-awareness—not to mention self-care—began back in college with the unconditional support of his coach. Instead of focusing on a number on the scale, his coach helped him quantify his health in a more self-loving manner by working toward goals of increased strength, speed, and performance. "I saw as I got healthier that my run times were coming down," Myles recalls. "This helped me eat more. I wanted to be healthy again. I wanted to feel strong."

Myles's road to healthy behavior hasn't been without hiccups. "So many evenings were spent in tears, even over the tiniest things—like meals I'd have to eat to remain properly fueled. But I eventually began to see how eating and gaining weight correlated with me being faster, which was a healthier focus for me in terms of my health."

Ultimately, the same coach who helped steer Myles away from self-destruction broached the possibility that he consider competing in athletic events, now that his strength had been renewed. Noting the speed with which he could run, the fluidity with which he swam, and the ease with which he took to cycling, she suggested he begin training for a triathlon. "Having overcome so much, I was ready for a new challenge," Myles says. He'd been living a balanced life after graduating from college and was considering graduate school. Aware that working toward athletic goals with a trustworthy team of coaches would bolster his attention to self-care and adequate nutrition—and having progressed greatly as an amateur athlete in between a day job in finance and an enjoyable social life—Myles decided to take his training to the next level. By 2013 he landed a spot as a triathlete on Team USA.

Myles's life today is packed. Each day begins around 4:30 am, when he kicks off his training by swimming, followed by breakfast, then a run at a nearby track or trail. If he feels up for it, he'll spin out his legs on a bike or do technique work (think: swimming, running, and cycling drills). Next up is lunch, another three-hour bike ride, and a carbohydrate-rich refueling snack (think: chocolate milk and oatmeal). Myles takes the next few hours to relax in a pair of medically engineered boots designed to flush lactic acid out of his legs by inflating with air, napping, then heading to the grocery store for the fruit, vegetables, and frequent pizza and/or pasta, which make up his dinner. After a hearty meal (and often a Netflix movie), Myles typically hits the hay around 7:00 pm.

When asked how his approach to exercise and eating today circumvents the definition of pathology, Myles points toward the motivations, results, and relative flexibility of his mind-set now as an answer. Rather than honing his bodily skills out of a compulsion, a sense of obligation, or a desire to be inhumanly thin, Myles sees his pursuit of athletic perfection as a meaningful endeavor from which he derives immense satisfaction. "I love my life. I can honestly say that," Myles remarks. "I don't feel I'm causing myself physical or psychological harm in my triathlon pursuit. I do it because I'm thrilled to." He's able to take time off when he needs it and he sees food as "fuel to live life, rather than something evil or bad, like I used to believe." To maintain self-awareness and to make sure he doesn't go over any emotional or physical edges, Myles regularly sees a therapist and closely follows the guidelines of his most trusted coach—his dad.

He also spends much of his downtime functioning as a National Eating Disorder Association navigator, offering support, guidance, and resources to individuals across the world struggling with body image and eating disturbances.

Most importantly, Myles has become highly aware of when he needs to increase his caloric intake to enhance his performance (or simply to recover) and he is no longer anxious about avoiding days off from training. "As my dad, also an athlete, has told me for years, 'You get faster when you're sitting on the couch.' It took me a while to get comfortable with the idea of resting. But now I see it as a part of my training—and a component of my overall health."

Retirement is a long way off for Myles, but when it comes time to ease back into a "civilian" exercise schedule, he plans on pursuing his PsyD. Myles dreams of one day becoming a therapist who specializes in—you guessed it!—body image issues, eating disturbances, and exercise addiction.

Myles's desire to reach out to individuals suffering in the shadows from anorexia, bulimia, or overzealous pursuits of fitness continues to grant his life purpose each day. "I felt so incredibly alone for so long," he admits. "I know there are thousands of people just like me out there, struggling silently. They need to know that there are others who have come out on the other side of their disorder. I wish I could tell them that they *can* get through it. Like me, they can go on to live a happy, healthy lifestyle."

JENNIFER HICKS

As a child, Jennifer abhorred exercise. "I was always very clumsy," she recalls of her earliest years. "I wasn't a little, thin, running-around-the-sports-field kind of girl. Anything physical felt uncomfortable to me."

Jennifer's primary focus was academia. She sidelined most types of physical fitness in favor of exercising her brain throughout most of her young adult life. It wasn't until she neared her late twenties that she gave running a go—in part, as a means to look her best in a wedding dress she anticipated donning after getting engaged to her college sweetheart, Paul, but also as an alternative strategy to manage the anxiety she'd combated for decades.

Jennifer's father committed suicide when she was barely three years old. Discussion of his death—and the unhappiness that led him to take his own life—was infrequent in her household. Jennifer recalls being encouraged to hide her true emotions, especially those that indicated any hint of sadness. "Emotions were a taboo where I grew up," Jennifer says. "I was taught—in large part, by the church I attended in girlhood—to believe crying made you a 'sinner.' I was terrified to emote at all, for fear of being judged." For years Jennifer worked tirelessly to swallow her feelings, channeling her focus into academic performance, intellectual prowess, and success in her coursework. No sooner had she graduated with a bachelor's degree in psychology and linguistics than she went on to pursue a graduate degree in speech-language pathology. "Basically, I had no life," Jennifer says. "My self-worth was tied to academia."

Despite her success in helping clients surmount communication issues once she'd landed a full-time position in her chosen profession, Jennifer's self-proclaimed perfectionist tendencies gradually extended to her pre-wedding fitness regimen. Having long internalized body image issues, she enjoyed the enhanced self-esteem and weight loss that becoming active entailed. Her running habits burgeoned from a few times a week to each day to multiple times per day. Jennifer insisted upon being physically active when spending time with her friends— dinners or movies, which required extended periods of sitting quickly became anathema to her—and quality time with her husband was consumed by her growing desire to put interpersonal connection on hold in favor of working out. She started carrying weights nearly everywhere she went, and even while driving to a romantic getaway for her honeymoon insisted on doing crunches, leg lifts, and other calorie-burning calisthenics in the car. "I was so anxious I couldn't sit still," Jennifer says. Her fixation on fitness became so engulfing that eventually she felt that she could not function without it. Jennifer even began lying to her husband about where she was going, pretending to be at a coffee shop for a few hours when really she was out jogging. She'd also drag him along on lengthy walks to destinations they both had in mind, trying to convince him wherever they were going was "just a short walk around the corner" when their destination was actually miles away. Like many exercise addicts, Jennifer's sleep suffered severely as a consequence of her obsessive thoughts related to working out, in addition to the early morning wakeups she'd endure in order to log enough time spent in motion before work.

At the height of her exercise addiction, Jennifer watched helplessly as her willpower to engage in basic acts of self-care (think: showering) fell by the wayside. She began going to work in her exercise clothing, inviting the concerned and confused attention of coworkers who worried for her health. Jennifer would learn later that many people in her professional and personal life had strong worries about her behavior, despite the fact that they refrained from pointing it out. "People all around me were disturbed by my behavior," she recalls, "but nobody really pointed it out. At work I was rapidly losing weight but no one was saying anything. So I just assumed my behavior was normal."

Eventually, however, Jennifer could no longer remain willfully unaware of the toll her overzealous physical activity habits were taking on her health. Her boss ultimately intervened to advise her to take a medical leave, a humiliating experience Jennifer describes as "horrifying."

Yet even this blow to her pride, which temporarily severed the connection to professionalism and career-based accomplishments that had so long kept her ego afloat, did not galvanize Jennifer to reduce her exercise routines. To the shock of most of her family members and friends, Jennifer instead impulsively sold her car to finance a trip to India for several months. "I was not well," Jennifer says of her mind-set during this time.

Her husband insisted on accompanying her so as to ensure her safety. Ultimately, the couple shared many enjoyable and illuminating moments—from a trip to the Taj Mahal to yoga lessons from a revered swami who taught them to do headstands. But once their departure date arrived, Jennifer insisted on staying. "I didn't know what I was looking for there but I knew, at the very least, I couldn't exercise to the extent that I had been prior to arriving." Desperate to be rescued from herself and the environment back home that she felt triggered her behavior, Jennifer convinced her husband to trust her instinct to remain in India while he flew back to their home in Toronto. She bounced around between Dharamasala and Rishikesh for weeks until she felt ready to leave.

Both during her time in India and prior to her extended trip, Jennifer had grappled with intrusive thoughts of suicide. Numerous times back home she considered jumping from a bridge that spanned a highway not far from the house where she lived with her husband. And during her overseas trip she knowingly drank unclean tap water and ate produce off the street, disregarding her awareness that such habits can lead to severe illness. "I was going about this in an almost passive suicidal way, as if to make myself sick," Jennifer recalls. Miraculously, Jennifer was spared from disease. She was also incredibly fortunate to run into a woman ten years her senior who happened to share some of Jennifer's history. "She knew what was going on with me," Jennifer reflects on the surprising overlaps of their behavioral patterns, "and she gave me a little bit of tough love. She called me out on a lot of my bullshit. It turned out to be really helpful. I learned a lot from her. All of what she taught me came from a place of her having had similar experiences to mine—addictions and all the rest of it!"

Time away from her home environment and immersion in a world where she couldn't engage in her regular habits of self-destruction—along with the support of an unexpected friend—helped Jennifer to reconsider her purpose and interest in life. About a month after her husband had arrived back in Toronto, she followed suit, enrolling herself in a training program to learn how to teach Nia technique classes—a practice a former coworker had introduced her to back when she was working full-time as a speech pathologist.

Initially, Jennifer saw the program as a means to enable her continuation of constant activity. After all, she figured, the combination of martial arts and dance that Nia incorporated was bound to burn numerous calories and keep her moving day in and day out. But even during her first training class, Jennifer's exercise-addicted mind-set was challenged. "It took me by surprise," she recalls. "Suddenly I was being asked to sense my body—how it felt when I placed my foot on the floor; how my hip felt when I moved a certain way. I was shocked. It felt so much better than pounding on pavement for hours on end like I was used to."

Though she was fairly skeptical about Nia's emphasis on keeping in touch with her own body's comfort levels, over time this novel approach to exercise began making more sense to her. "When I first started teaching, I had to pretend that I was comfortable in my body—because it took some time before I really was. But I feel that in pretending I actually learned how to be okay in my skin—how to feel confident about myself." Jennifer doesn't recall the process as easy. "I had no physical background," she admits, recalling her aversion to most types of exercise from an early age. "So to be teaching dance was way out of my comfort zone."

Coupled with her teaching, Jennifer sought the help of a psychiatrist who helped her to find a viable medication regimen that granted her a newfound peace of mind. Accepting that she should take medication took almost as much effort as wrenching her mind-set out of obsession. But eventually, she began to see how such treatment rendered her more functional. She was relieved at finding a treatment that ultimately worked for her, as she'd spent years struggling to comprehend most eating disorder treatment facilities' insistence on ceasing exercise entirely, being monitored to an extent that negated her privacy, and subjecting her to what she felt was "a militaristic approach to 'getting better' that just shut me down."

The combination of a prescription that agreed with her, a renewed awareness in her body through her Nia instruction, and the new community of people she met through her work who modeled healthier views about their own bodies and exercise habits gradually brought Jennifer back from the brink. She went on to found her own business—once again practicing speech therapy in addition to her Nia teaching—and mustered the courage to explore her creative side, an aspect of her personality she feels she'd stifled for too many years. Jennifer regularly journals, writes professionally, and makes collages. These outlets not only provide her a regular dose of fun, but they also enable her to communicate those thoughts and feelings that she still occasionally struggles to put into words. When not dancing, working with speech pathology clients, or putting her all into one of her chosen creative endeavors, Jennifer enjoys the company of her husband and her new group of friends. She also functions as a mental health advocate. "My whole lifestyle is different," Jennifer says, comparing her daily existence today to her former obligatory slog of tireless self-punishment through exercise. "I'm so much more social now than I used to be, even if I do still consider myself an introvert. I listen to myself now—I tune into what I need. I surround myself with good people, my relationship with my husband is strong, and I'm so satisfied with my work." Jennifer has also come far in terms of getting better in touch with her emotions. "My husband and my twin sister used to call me the 'tin woman' because of how cut off I was from my emotions. Now I'm much more aware. If I can't actually say what I'm feeling, I'll figure it out in writing. I'll tell my husband, 'read this; this is what's going on with me.' That's new. It's taken me a long time to not feel shame around my emotions."

Jennifer no longer feels compelled to exercise to the extent that her body and mind suffer. Although the nature of her job keeps her on her feet more than the average North American, Jennifer sees her current relationship to physical activity as healthy, healing, and enjoyable. Licking her addiction to working out wasn't about giving up exercise entirely, Jennifer notes. "It was about finding how to do this thing that helps me in a way that wasn't over the top. It was about learning to appreciate my body and find the pleasure and joy in movement—just as in life." Lucky for her students, this approach to fitness is precisely what they can hope to learn when taking one of her Nia classes.

"It's a daily practice," says Jennifer. "I'm so grateful to be in a position to teach what I need to learn—that our bodies are wonderful and they deserve to be treated with respect."

MARION MACLEAN

Following the lead of her older and younger brothers, Marion Maclean, the middle child of three kids, recalls playing just about every sport imaginable throughout grade school. Marion was raised in an extremely active household, encouraged by her father to pursue sports after school and on weekends so as to stay off the streets of a formerly dangerous hometown.

She excelled in virtually all of her attempts at athleticism (football included), raking in trophies, awards, and placing first in running and swimming competitions throughout high school. At age fifteen, Marion put sports on hold to take up a job that ate up her free time with its long hours and lengthy commute.

Living in this community of athletes gave her a sense of belonging, boosted her self-esteem, and offered her a healthy outlet that improved her physical and emotional well-being. At the outset, Marion considered her relationship to physical activity to be very normal. Only after she removed herself from this world and delved into work did she find herself slowly beginning to obsess over exercise.

Marion was sixteen when she met her future first husband, Tony, a bodybuilder, who encouraged her to join him each day at the gym. Marion quickly took to aerobics classes, progressing from two per week to daily sessions that totaled forty hours a week at the peak of her exercise addiction.

Contributing to this time spent in motion was Marion's additional schedule as a fitness instructor. Having fallen in love with the classes offered by her local gym, she pursued accreditation to share the joy she felt and to teach others, motivated by "the hype and atmosphere of all the beautiful people lunging, jumping, kicking, and twisting to a fast-paced musical beat." Prior to her wedding Marion started to feel self-conscious about a small amount of weight she'd put on. But Marion found satisfaction from the effects this extra workload of fitness had upon her physique. "I loved the attention it delivered and it seemed to make Tony proud," Marion recalls. "All of this boosted my ego and sent my self-esteem soaring. Before long, I was captivated by the whole idea of the gym world."

It wasn't long before she started pursuing bodybuilding in addition to teaching aerobics and working full-time—eventually competing at the professional lightweight level. An obsession had begun but Marion was oblivious. "My days, nights, and months at the gym rolled into one unbroken cycle of training," she recalls.

A typical day for her during this time started at 6:30 am, where she'd take a few personal training clients under her wing prior to guiding gym-goers through multiple high-impact aerobics classes. Instead of taking a break following her morning's exertion, Marion would go on to instruct weight classes and then work on honing her own musculature well into the evening. She'd take on a few more personal training clients after work hours, hopping into yet another aerobics class just before dinnertime.

Reflecting on the height of her addiction, Marion emphasizes how powerful an overzealous obsession with fitness can be: "Exercise addiction drastically affects the whole purpose of your life. From the first minute you wake up, you start obsessing over the plan for the day's training. You're unable to have a conversation about any subject other than training." Marion was psychologically trapped in a relentless cycle of continual acceleration in her cardio routines and increased intensity of her weight-lifting sessions. Friends, family, and rationality fell by the wayside as Marion's focus was on her need to train.

Though Marion can't put a finger on a single reason undergirding her addictive zeal for working out, she has a strong hunch that its roots tie to her yearnings for attention, approval, and a sense of belonging—exacerbated, in large part, by her institutionalization as a child (beginning at age four) in the wake of her mother's suicide. Add to this her first husband's disparaging comments about her postmarriage weight gain, and she believes this triggered "an eventual journey to a much darker place." Though Marion miraculously incurred only minor physical injuries as a result of her relentless training regimen, her mental stability was devastatingly damaged. Before long, Marion's behavior led her to suffer a nervous breakdown.

After hitting an emotional rock bottom, Marion sought counseling to alleviate the dangerous thought process that had left her in psychological disarray. Marion's life spiraled down into the absolute depths of despair, losing her marriage and nearly losing her life. With the help of family and friends, Marion saw a glimmer of light at the end of the dark tunnel that would eventually lead her to researching and educating herself about eating disorders and pathological relationships with physical activity. Though she explains it took many years to reroute her mind and body toward a more self-respectful and healthier perspective—"the recovery did not happen overnight," she says, "nor did it involve never again thinking about weight, exercise, or body image." Marion gradually achieved a more balanced, rational view of exercise. With help, she learned to replace "negative self-critical thoughts with positive, affirmative ones" and practiced exercising "in a non-competitive, non-obsessive way."

Marion cites eating disorder activist Carolyn Costin and motivational speaker Paul Hanna as inspirations to her recovery, along with a serendipitous image of survival that she happened upon during an impromptu shopping trip. "One day, I saw a cartoon of a frog about to be swallowed in a pelican's beak," Marion remembers. "Even in his almost terminal situation, the frog had one arm free and was trying to choke the pelican so he could not be swallowed. The caption read "Never, ever give up." When I got home I wrote "Never, Never, Never, Give Up" on my bathroom mirror, and I committed myself with a diamond-hard conviction to explore the reasons behind my illness. I threw myself into research, devouring everything I could find on eating or exercise disorders. The more I learned, the more I understood about my own obsessive phases and subsequent decline into depression."

Though painstaking in her pursuit of recovery, Marion highlights the often-frustrating length of time reorienting her mind toward self-help rather than self-harm took. "Even with the support of my friends and family, my full recovery took years. It had to start with minuscule flashes of recognition that I had a problem. Then through research, I'd have a flash of insight into what the causes might have been," she says.

Marion now avoids the gym. Her busy schedule working as a sport and recreation coach, providing physical activity programs for children, teenagers, and adults with intellectual, physical, and sensory disabilities, keeps her moving around enough. Marion also functions as a care worker for these clients, helping to inclusively integrate them into their communities. "I like to think at the end of my busy day that I made some small contribution to enhancing a client's quality of life," Marion says of a job she finds deeply satisfying.

Her preferred physical activity these days is walking. But though she shoots for a goal of thirty minutes at a brisk pace, she doesn't speed down sidewalks or up trails out of compulsion. Rather, she walks to keep her heart and lungs healthy, in the interest of supporting the cardiovascular system she hopes to keep strong for her future grandchildren. Marion is the proud mother of a thirteen-year-old daughter, Alana, and she's pleased to report she's been happily remarried for fourteen years.

8

WHAT TO DO ABOUT IT

Treatment

Exercise addicts may seek treatment when an injury prevents them from continuing their preferred routines, when a loved one urges them to consult a therapist, or when the rigidity of their fitness schedules becomes emotionally or physically unmanageable. If the physical aches and pains that their overzealous cardiovascular or weight-lifting habits introduce into their lives end up restricting the range of exercises they can perform, they may be galvanized to seek therapy simply to manage the severe emotional turmoil (and ego crisis) accompanying a forced reduction in the activity that they so pathologically cherish.

Whether one or several stress fractures prompts a reconsideration of whether their workouts are safe or whether a series of failed relationships causes them to question whether their running schedule is hampering their hopes of finding a life partner, many exercise addicts inevitably are confronted by their disorder's unmistakable intrusion upon the rest of their lives. Anxiety, depression, or relational and professional conflicts inspired by excessive exercise can be the tipping point for some sufferers to reach out for help, even if they may not fully recognize the contribution of their relentless workouts to many of their personal and social woes. Others may seek the guidance of a therapist upon realizing their behavior has spun out of control, out of fear that they may irreversibly hurt themselves or from a state of desperation to re-spark what they once knew as life outside of the gym.

The research into *why* a primary or secondary exercise addict seeks treatment is, at best, scant. Even more limited are the number of studies testing the outcomes of therapies targeted specifically toward overzealous physical activity. Because exercise addiction is such a novel concept in the field of mental health—keep in mind even the American Psychiatric Association has not included exercise addiction, among other behavioral addictions, as a legitimate disorder in its *Diagnostic and Statistical Manual of Mental Disorders*—there simply hasn't been as much time and information to develop specialized treatments for it as there has been for other disorders, like eating pathologies or substance dependency.

There's no pat prescription that'll guarantee an instantaneous recovery from being hooked on the gym, and there isn't a magic pill one can take to "cure" the disorder. But there are a number of treatment options of which exercise addicts can take advantage that have been shown to ameliorate the symptoms of other behavioral addictions as well as the symptoms of eating disorders.

Under extreme circumstances when an exercise addict's behavior has put his or her own physical health at risk—as can be the case with secondary exercise addiction, when severe food restriction accompanies overzealous activity or when an addict's bodily systems begin breaking down in response to acute or chronic overexertion—inpatient treatment may be advised.

Some exercise addicts may also willfully opt for inpatient treatment if they feel they need to be temporarily removed from the environments in which their addiction initially started. Taking a medical leave to kick-start their recovery may appeal to those individuals who prefer a more structured and monitored venue in which they can learn, practice, and implement a healthier approach to exercise. There are currently no inpatient programs specifically designed to treat exercise addiction alone. However, many eating disorder treatment facilities address pathological relationships with physical activity in their approaches. (For a list of these facilities, please refer to appendix A.)

Oftentimes when nutritional restriction accompanies an exercise addict's daily routines, the first step in treatment is stabilizing his or her weight. More often than not, this involves temporary abstention from all physical activity until scale numbers reach healthier levels. Not surprisingly, most (secondary) exercise addicts balk at this common attempt to reverse or stem the physical damage incurred by compulsive overexercise coupled with undernourishment. But a growing body of evidence suggests their resistance may not be entirely unfounded. While secondary exercise addicts undoubtedly need to be cleared by a physician before participating in physical activity (just as anyone with any health condition would be) maintaining a fitness regimen throughout their recovery process is by no means an insurmountable impediment to resuming a healthy weight. As long as the secondary exercise addict adequately refuels to compensate for lost calories—in the beginning stages of regaining weight, this may mean doubling or tripling their typical daily caloric intake—physical activities can be sustained. In fact, there's even proof that maintaining a moderate exercise schedule may help ameliorate eating-disordered symptoms.[1] Unfortunately, many well-intentioned approaches to treating eating disorders in those who use exercise in self-destructive ways have ignored the many ways in which moderate activity can contribute to physical recovery and mental health.

When engaged in reasonably, willfully, and spontaneously (rather than out of compulsion, as a means of self-punishment, or as an alternate method of purging), exercise lowers the risk factors for eating-disordered behaviors. Despite concerns that it may perpetuate, contribute to, or hinder a person's recovery from eating-disordered behavior, normal levels of physical activity have been proven to be perfectly safe for those trying to overcome anorexia, bulimia, and all unhealthy food-related habits in between.[2]

With the right mind-set, keeping active reduces depression and anxiety, lifts negative moods, enhances body image, and improves self-esteem. It can also help ease the uncomfortable bodily responses to the re-feeding process that anorexic individuals must undergo as part of their treatment, along with alleviating the bloating and distention even non-eating-disordered individuals experience after meals. What's more, sticking to a moderate fitness regimen has been shown to enhance self-regulation—a skill that just about anyone can benefit from honing, especially those who struggle with self-harm and addiction. And maintaining an active lifestyle helps rescue those prone to social isolation from walling themselves off inside an unhealthy spiral of self-destruction. Perhaps most importantly for those who are underweight, exercise (especially strength training) aids the resumption of a healthy BMI by helping to increase muscle mass.

Exercise addicts can be incredibly resistant to treatment, as some of them may equate receiving care with losing the superhuman discipline and independence they've worked so strenuously to cultivate prior to seeking help.

Underweight or not, overzealous exercisers who hope to break the addictive cycle of self-destructive physical activity levels may benefit from a finite respite from their over-the-top habits. Whether this break from exercise spans a few days, a week, or several months, temporary abstention is crucial to recalibrating the body's mental and physiological balance as well as to bringing to the surface those anxieties and fears which undergird the exercise addict's compulsive pursuit of fitness.

Ideally, both primary and secondary recovering exercise addicts can work closely with behavioral addiction specialists or therapists well versed in eating disorders to process the emotional turmoil that surges in response to dialing back their routines and exploring what lies beneath their compulsions to continually remain in motion. If they can afford to work with a fitness professional (i.e., a personal trainer) who is properly trained to recognize and comprehend unhealthy habits at the gym, all the better. Since many individuals who work in the fitness industry are themselves physically in shape, this may enable the exercise addict to be less wary of their advice to slow down, rest, and adequately refuel as needed. Many exercise addicts struggle to trust that another person's advice to reduce their routines comes from an informed and knowledgeable place.

As one secondary exercise addict puts it,

> it's a scary thing when you have to be told that your approach to exercise is, well, crazy. When you suffer from a compulsion to over-exercise you're so set in your ways—you think you understand every-thing about building muscle and burning fat. So much of it is about control. But you can't get past your problem without giving up some of that control. It was really difficult but eventually I started to see that the professionals whose job it was to help me recover—the doctors, the therapists, even my coach—didn't have any ulterior mo-tives. I think the hardest thing to trust is that there is no great con-spiracy, no one's trying to make you obese. They're just trying to help. And you have to let go a little and let them.

The goal of any exercise addict's journey to recovery is to learn what a feasible amount of physical activity feels like—and to recover the initial pleasure they once derived from exercise. Rather than the anxiety-provoking and compulsive adherence to an overly fatiguing regimen that drove their body and mind into an untenable rut, the improved relationship to physical activity is characterized by feasibility and enjoyment. Feasibility needn't mean not challenging. Rather, a healthier fitness plan should fit smoothly into the recovering exercise addict's other life interests (and obligations), be flexible, as stress-free as possible, and, most importantly, fun.

Most recovering exercise addicts find that regular communication with therapists, trusted trainers, and/or knowledgeable loved ones about all the negative thoughts, feelings, and impulses that surface during the new routine aids in their self-awareness and mental ease. Keeping a journal or log to track the ebb, flow, and content of accompanying emotions and urges is also an option some former exercise addicts consider a boon to their well-being.

TREATMENT OPTIONS

Exercise addicts looking to overcome their struggles with overzealous fitness habits may want to explore a range of treatment options, chief among them cognitive behavioral therapy (CBT), acceptance and commitment therapy (ACT), medication, and alternative approaches such as nutraceuticals, mindfulness practices, and a more intuitive and natural approach to keeping fit. Although further research needs to be conducted to validate whether such approaches have an equally powerful effect on the symptoms of exercise addiction, that they have been proven effective in ameliorating a range of mood and behavioral issues—ranging from depression, anxiety, and impulsivity to eating disorders, substance dependence, and self-harm—makes them promising candidates for the treatment of exercise addiction.

A helpful approach in determining what type of treatment best suits an exercise addict is by identifying his or her stage of change. Outlined by psychologists James O. Prochaska and Carlo C. DiClemente in 1982,[3] these stages include precontemplation, contemplation, preparation, action, maintenance, and termination.

During the precontemplation stage, people are not ready to alter their behavior at all. Either they are too enmeshed in their current maladaptive behaviors or they're up against an overwhelming number of time and feasibility barriers that prevents them from conceiving how they might alter their habits. Contemplation, by contrast, means considering a shift in how they act. They are thinking about changing their behavior, shifting from "I will not" or "I cannot" to "Well, I might. . . ." During preparation, people are beginning to slowly introduce changes into their behavior, albeit not enough to fully overcome their previously self-destructive inclinations. Action entails changing the behavior—or surmounting whatever bad habit had previously engulfed them. Relapse is common during the preparation and action stages because the new behavior is not fully ingrained. Maintenance, the end result of repeated attempts to prevail through setbacks along the path to behavioral change, is the continued commitment to the new mode of living.

It is critical for therapists to conduct motivational interviews with new clients whom they suspect may suffer from exercise addiction so as to determine their current stage on the behavioral change model.

For any exercise addict entertaining the possibility that he or she might have a problem with a supposedly healthy behavior, ambivalence about committing to treatment will likely be high. Trained therapists must do their best, therefore, to identify this hesitancy and highlight the imbalance between negative and positive consequences brought about by their patients' extreme engagements in overexertion. The more exercise addicts become aware of how their compulsive physical activity patterns markedly decrease their quality of life, the more willing they can become to remapping their behavior and thought patterns with the help of a trusted mental health professional.[4]

A significant force in exercise addicts' compulsive behavior is a fixation on self-mastery—be it over the body or of the time spent exercising, the distance run, the calories burned, the pounds lifted, or the reps completed. This fixation may border on delusion, inasmuch as the exercise addict has, by definition, lost control over his or her behavior, and many treatments may be, at first, heavily resisted by the exercise addict as they require him or her to cede some degree of agency in order to be helped. The prospect of altering behavior may provoke a great deal of anxiety in the exercise addict, who may predicate the strength and stability of his or her identity upon each daily gym session. That those much-coveted workouts help the exercise addict cope with everything from boredom to broken body images renders the thought of making more time for other activities seem initially insurmountable—if not downright depressing. After all, even nonaddicted exercisers who work out frequently experience dips in mood on days they can't get to the gym (even if those dips don't precipitate mood swings, irritability, or hamper their ability to focus on other tasks, as it would for exercise addicts).

To help ease fitness addicts' reluctance to alter their schedules and warm them to the possibility of change, some therapists recommend emphasizing to compulsively exercising clients how much control they are actively taking over their disorder by seeking help—thereby clarifying for patients that they are (rightly) maintaining (albeit rerouting) their much-sought-after autonomy and independence.

Cognitive Behavioral Therapy

The techniques of cognitive behavioral therapy (CBT) may be useful in treating the symptoms of exercise addiction. Like drug addicts or alcoholics, exercise addicts can work with a trained cognitive behavioral therapist to monitor and explore those faulty thought patterns that lead them to exercise in a pathological manner. Cognitive behavioral therapists can also work with exercise addicts to further examine their deeply ingrained beliefs about the body as well as the meaning behind their relentless physical activity. Keep in mind that there are currently no definitive studies directly linking CBT's treatment outcomes to the recovery from exercise addiction. However, CBT techniques have been shown to be effective in treating the symptoms of anorexia nervosa, binge eating disorder, and bulimia,[5] along with anxiety,[6] substance use disorders,[7] and other behavioral addictions[8] (i.e., compulsive gambling, compulsive spending, and sex addiction).

A large part of CBT involves challenging what the patient believes to be true—that is, *I cannot survive without my daily two (or more) hour workouts* or *I am less valuable as a person if I am not constantly improving my physique*. Clients' assumptions are reframed as hypotheses that require evidence in order to be proven. Exercise addicts may be prompted by cognitive behavioral therapists to "verify" a deeply held sense that they are worthless or nonfunctional in the absence of their preferred workout regimen—say, for example, by participating in another activity, by cutting back on the gym for a short period of time, or by offering a valid argument to prove their supposed worthlessness (hint: the chances they'll come up with a rational justification? Slim to none).

When a behavioral shift is implemented (most often a reduction in activity or a change in the time or nature of activity an exercise addict engages in), CBT clients can discuss the feelings and concerns that crop up during each therapy session. CBT patients will often be asked to keep a journal or log of the instinctive, negative thoughts that spring into their minds when access to exercise is limited. Most CBT patients also receive homework assignments to complete outside therapy hours—for example, listing goals, weighing pros and cons of each goal, creating agendas for subsequent therapy sessions, completing assigned reading, itemizing knee-jerk assumptions, and attempting to find data to prove or disprove those assumptions.

The goal of CBT in the context of exercise addiction is not to prevent the client from ever working out again, but instead to learn how to recognize from where the negative thoughts arise that fuel the addictive behavior (as well as how to stop them in their tracks before they consume the exercise addict and tip her back into a self-destructive activity pattern).

Patients are typically rewarded for abstaining from or reducing the amount of self-abusive exercise in which they engage (per an agreed-upon plan that the patient and therapist develop throughout the therapeutic program), thus easing the obsessive need to master the body while maladaptive beliefs (i.e., that exercise is *always* a good idea, no matter how compulsively or hurtfully it's performed) are ironed out during each therapy session.

CBT is well suited not only to recovering addicts who are looking for time-sensitive (albeit obviously not immediate) results but also to those who seek wallet-friendly approaches. Many CBT therapists take insurance, and the typical duration of CBT ranges from twelve to twenty weeks—if not four to eight weeks, to accommodate limited schedules.[9]

A common assignment for CBT clients is keeping a "thought record" that accounts for situations; automatic thoughts, emotions, and moods; evidence to support those thoughts; evidence to disprove those thoughts; and alternative (read: more logical and rational) thoughts.

Clients may also be asked to keep track of automatic behaviors, antecedents to those behaviors, and the long- and short-term consequences of their knee-jerk reactions to stress.

Charlotte Andersen, who we met in the last chapter, believes CBT was the pivot point in her ability to move beyond unhealthy exercise habits. Her therapist had her write down all the repetitive thoughts she had—that is, "I only like myself when I'm working out" and "No one will love me if I get fat." With her therapist, Charlotte generated reasonable rebuttals to those all-or-nothing cognitive distortions—think: "I'm not going to gain fifty pounds overnight if I don't get to the gym" and "Everyone misses a day here or there! It's okay to take time off!" Though she admits it was incredibly difficult to believe these corrections at the outset of her therapy, within weeks she was already noticing a difference.

Charlotte combined these strategies with a close cousin of CBT, exposure response prevention therapy (ERPT). With this approach, Charlotte set goals with her therapist, like scheduling one less workout a week or going to the gym and reading a book in the lobby to practice quelling the anxiety-ridden compulsion to overexercise. "I would do these things and realize that I'd done them—and that it was okay. I survived." Over time, Charlotte gathered enough experience and evidence to disprove her assumptions that she couldn't function without her rigid and overly rigorous exercise schedule. "It was the smallest change," she says, "just a little rewording on my thoughts. But it had the biggest effect. For the first time I was finally treating my underlying issues rather than just changing my physical behavior." As Charlotte began understanding how illogical her thought patterns were, the panic and compulsiveness surrounding her activities dialed down remarkably.

Medications

The data on pharmacological approaches to ameliorating exercise addiction is scarce. One study suggests antipsychotics may help lower the severity of sufferers' symptoms. (Four weeks into a daily regimen of quetiapine—an antipsychotic drug used to treat schizophrenia, bipolar disorder, and depression—one addict saw his urge to compulsively exercise dwindle. Within twenty-four weeks, his compulsions to engage in obsessive patterns of physical activity had become virtually nonexistent.[10])

Other studies examining the impact of medication on symptoms of eating disorders[11] and non-exercise-related addictive behaviors (i.e., Internet addiction and pathological gambling) suggest serotonin reuptake inhibitors, mood stabilizers, and some anti-dependence drugs[12] may assist sufferers with symptom management. Since anxiety is often an influential component of exercise addiction, antianxiety medications may also be prescribed. Far more research into pharmaceutical treatment of compulsive exercise is required, however, before a valid consensus can be reached about what medication options best suit exercise addicts. Each individual seeking treatment must confer on a case-by-case basis with a psychiatrist to determine whether pharmaceutical intervention is appropriate and, if so, which kind will work best.

Nutraceuticals

Because many exercise addicts are health conscious, they may be more amenable to natural medicinal approaches to managing their mood and behavioral issues. Some studies have reported that supplementation with vitamins C and E and other antioxidants such as resveratrol[13, 14] can reduce symptoms or indicators of the oxidative stress that naturally results from exercise. Exercise appears to increase reactive oxygen species (i.e., free radicals), which can damage the body's cells. The antioxidant-exercise hypothesis is simple: exercise more, breathe more, oxidize more. So the idea of boosting the antioxidant reserves to offset the perceived negative effects of exercise emerged. Those who subject their bodies to excessive exercise might have an increased need for natural means of resolving the damage brought about by overzealous activity.

As far as mood is concerned, the spice saffron (from the indigenous southwest Asian plant *Crocus sativus L.*) has emerged as a promising herbal compound for the treatment of depression and for generally boosting mood. Similar to antidepressants, saffron may modulate the levels of certain chemicals in the brain, including serotonin. Although it has been proposed that saffron increases serotonin levels in the brain, the exact mechanism of action for this is unknown. A recent meta-analysis[15] found that saffron supplementation was just as effective as antidepressants in improving the mood of patients with major depression.

Because nutraceuticals are not regulated by the FDA, consumers must research the supplements they want to buy to ensure that they are high quality (read: that they contain no added fillers). All-natural versions produced through good manufacturing practice are available along with clinical studies to support their proclaimed health benefits.

Acceptance and Commitment Therapy

An alternative approach to treating exercise addiction is acceptance and commitment therapy (ACT).[16] ACT involves training a patient to come to terms with those uncomfortable feelings and inevitable frustrations that would normally precipitate impulses to run to the gym—rather than, say, to sit with—read: tolerate—unease. ACT has been empirically shown to help manage symptoms of anxiety[17] and has proven particularly effective in the treatment of eating disorders[18] and depression.[19]

A core component of ACT involves cognitive diffusion, the mental skill of identifying emotions or thoughts for what they are (i.e., temporarily overwhelming) rather than what we fear they might be (say, interminably unmanageable). For the exercise addict this might mean re-evaluating fears that a missed gym session will mean a dissolution of identity and worth (via loss of muscle, loss of strength, or gaining weight). Acceptance that taking a day (or more) off is healthy rather than harmful—or that a transient loss of strength or stamina due to extended time off does not pose a risk to the exercise addict's human integrity and value as a person—would be another example of how ACT might be incorporated into a recovering exercise addict's therapy regimen.

Ultimately, the goal of ACT is to work away from avoidance-based negative coping styles and toward acknowledgment and acceptance of difficulties, setbacks, and shortcomings.

Meditation

Mindfulness, meditation, and other self- and body-awareness exercises have also been incredibly effective in the treatment of eating disorders[20]—not to mention a host of other mental health issues ranging from depression[21] to substance abuse[22] and even psychosis.[23]

Although research hasn't definitively linked meditation to the amelioration of exercise addiction symptoms per se, numerous studies have confirmed the practice's positive effect on reducing stress, anxiety, and a range of compulsive urges. One study,[24] for example, found that three months of weekly basic breathing exercises helped adults alleviate their obsessive-compulsive disorder symptoms and enhanced their sense of purpose in life.

In general, yoga—the relaxed, mindful kind, not the kind that encourages practitioners to push themselves beyond their body's limits of endurance or flexibility—has been shown to positively augment anxiousness and its accompanying stress hormones.[25] Exercise addicts might do well to take up a moderate yoga practice under the guidance of a teacher who emphasizes self-awareness and respect for the body over physical perfection in poses.

Psychoeducation

Research suggests[26] that psychoeducation is a core component of moving beyond exercise addiction. The discussion of feasible goals for one's body, rational (read: healthy) body image, adequate and proper nutrition, and literacy in responding to media images promoting thinness, muscularity, or fitness has been shown to be incredibly helpful to recovering exercise addicts. Often, workoutaholics enter treatment with inhumanly high expectations of themselves along with unrealistic standards that, being impossible to meet, relentlessly erode their self-esteem each time they fail to meet them.

Some psychologists[27] encourage imparting the classical psychological concept of reciprocal determinism to patients suffering from exercise addiction. Reciprocal determinism, as coined and conceived by Alfred Bandura in 1986, posits that our behavior influences the environment in which we exist and that this environment loops back to influence our thoughts and feelings. Therefore, Bandura believed, any change we make to one of these three entities (thoughts, behaviors, or environment) will inevitably affect the other two. If the exercise addict can understand that changing her environment will help change her thoughts about exercise as well as the behaviors she engages in as a reaction to those thoughts, she may be more amenable to undergoing treatment—say, by removing herself from the gym she belongs to or by scheduling a therapy session during the time that she'd normally spend working out, so as to begin chipping away at the obsessive urge to build more muscle, log more miles, or remain in motion that prompts her to spend upward of three hours each day at the gym.

Exercise Reprogramming

Many treatment facilities help train compulsive exercisers to relearn what exercising in a healthier way feels like. Techniques offered by the likes of Monte Nido, the Rader Program, Linden Oaks, La Ventana, and other inpatient and outpatient programs across the United States and Canada (see the list of facilities in appendix A) not only expose patients to the behavior that provokes such anxiety to begin with (thereby guiding them through panic in order to practice calmness in the face of triggers), but they also work with clients to practice moderate amounts of physical activities ranging from low-impact routines like yoga or pilates to more strenuous ones such as weight training; reasonable amounts of jogging, biking, or swimming; and some types of dance. The goal of incorporating exercise into treatment plans for inpatient and outpatient programs is—after securing medical clearance and ensuring that a patient's weight is at a level stable enough to engage in regular exercise—to retrain individuals to move in ways that *feel good* to them both mentally and physically rather than in ways that stem from self-punishment, anxiety-provoking guilt, or compulsion.

"My job is not to make my clients couch potatoes," explains Angie Lockwood, a nurse and fitness trainer at Monte Nido's Agoura Hills, California, location. "It's to make exercise *add* to their lives again rather than taking away from who they are. Exercise is supposed to make your life better, not make you a slave.

"We want to experiment with exercise while they're in treatment. We don't want them to leave without any guidance or support surrounding their use of the gym."

Lockwood remarks on the powerful shift in focus that occurs when her clients learn to incorporate a variety of activities into their lives in a flexible manner. "The cardio queens who come in seem to calm down a bit with the weight training. It seems to change their mind-set from how much they run to how strong they can get. It's such a pleasure to be around them when they've come down off that frenetic place they walked in with. They are quieter. They listen more. It's really interesting and, quite frankly, kind of magical. There's such a remarkable change in the energy as they undergo treatment—that's pretty much across the board."

A large part of enabling this transition involves establishing trust. Trainers and therapists know this well from clients from all levels of physical fitness or psychological stability. Lockwood offers her own story as grounds for establishing a bond that allows patients to open up. "I, too, used to overexercise," she explains. "I was crazy—I exercised through a herniated disc to a point where I almost lost the use of my left calf. I had to get surgery and I was on bed rest for six weeks! I tell this to my patients—I show them my scars—to get them to trust me. And when they do, that's when the changes begin to happen."

Other Approaches

Intuitive Exercise

Another approach to reintegrating a moderate amount of fitness into a former exercise addict's weekly schedule involves a relatively new take on fitness dubbed by some experts as "intuitive exercise."

Although discipline and commitment are inherent components of any fitness regimen, the philosophy of intuitive exercise is that physical activity should be driven by pleasure rather than by pain or suffering. (Think: exercising because you *want* to, not because you *have* to; pursuing activities that make you feel good and that you enjoy, rather than ones you detest and subject yourself to only because you've been told they're "good" for you.)

An intuitive exerciser opts for challenging and engaging workouts that he has fun doing and fundamentally likes. This is the opposite of the addictive exerciser who pursues activities based solely on how many calories he can expect to burn, how many miles he can log, or how much muscle he can build. The exercise addict's painstaking denial of his body's stop and slow-down signals differentiates him from the intuitive exerciser, who doesn't avoid rest periods and who listens to his body when his muscles and joints need a break.

The intuitive exerciser chooses movement patterns that fit her energy level, lifestyle, and body type—and she doesn't limit herself to a set number of rigid routines like an exercise addict does. Variation is key to the intuitive exerciser's approach to fitness, as is abandoning thoughts about fat, body shape, size, and calories while working out.

Neuromuscular Integrative Action (Nia) Technique

Synthesizing dance and martial arts (think: tae kwon do and tai chi), the Nia technique is a mindfulness-based and healing-oriented movement practice that some mental health professionals recommend to clients struggling with body image issues. Several former exercise addicts cite Nia as crucial to their recovery process, as the technique's encouragement of self-love, creativity, body awareness, and pleasure in movement (rather than pain) can help cultivate a more intuitive approach to exercise. In addition to improving body image, alleviating anxiety, and improving mood, many practitioners claim that Nia helps to alleviate chronic pain, improve flexibility, and enhance cardiovascular health.

MovNat

Developed by Erwan Le Corre as a means of revisiting how our ancestors used to move, MovNat emphasizes perfecting the body's basic abilities (think: climbing a tree, jumping, pulling up one's own body weight, crawling, and balancing). Occasionally confused with its more competitive cousin, CrossFit (also designed around mastering those physical movements our active ancestors supposedly did much better than us), MovNat claims to be more varied and less rigid. Exercise addicts obsessed with repeating an inflexible series of movements or with bulking up may do well to test MovNat's perspective, shifting away from isolating various muscle groups and fixating on burnt calories to learning how to move the body as a whole. Another emphasis from Le Corre's program: unplugging the iPod, the television, or whatever other distracting apparatus you use to get yourself through a workout and to focus on your body in motion. And as any MovNatter will tell you, this also involves taking your routine outdoors!

FURTHER SUGGESTIONS

Recovering exercise addicts may also want to reevaluate the kind of gym to which they belong. Many health clubs and fitness franchises promote pushing past pain, gunning toward superhuman levels of strength, or striving toward lower weights by burning more calories. Individuals with already extant body image and self-esteem issues—especially those prone to eating disorders—tend to be particularly sensitive to these campaigns and are more likely to incorporate such messages into their lives in a self-destructive manner.[28]

Merely looking at images of athletic and toned bodies has been shown to increase body dissatisfaction among males,[29] while women's body esteem scores plummet after viewing photos of slimmer same-sex models.[30, 31] Studies suggest that fitness trainers who focus far too much on their own body fat and muscularity also tend to have a negative impact on their clients' body image.[32]

Because cost can be a primary predictor of the gym to which you belong or where you have access to fitness equipment or cardiovascular training outlets, the recovering exercise addict's best bet is to ally himself with a trainer at the gym he frequents whom he feels comfortable confiding in and discussing triggers that launch him back into the addictive thought process. Needless to say, it is highly recommended that exercise addicts at all stages of their recovery process continue individual or group therapy until exercise can be engaged in safely without overwhelming urges to jump back into self-destructive patterns of movement.

Overwriting the neural pathways that have been continually reinforced through negative self-talk, self-abuse, and painstaking repetitions of excessive routines is no small task. Getting over exercise addiction won't happen overnight, nor can most exercise addicts accomplish recovery solely on their own. Accepting the help of others is a huge part of moving out of the addictive cycle, as many exercise addicts tend to negate their own human needs for love, self-care, and pleasure, all the while striving toward a nearly inhuman level of ostensible independence.[33]

Learning to approach physical activity from a place of self-care rather than self-abuse or obsession requires cultivating a sense of mastery of one's own ability to exercise in a healthy, non-self-destructive manner.

Important in the process of developing this mastery is the availability of role models or easily comprehensible and trustworthy examples of healthier exercise regimens. These models can include a personal trainer, fitness instructor, or close friend sensitive to the needs of an individual recovering from exercise addiction—someone who can both demonstrate and guide the exercise addict through more moderate, yet still challenging and engaging, exercise habits.

Therapists and fitness professionals sensitive to the needs of recovering exercise addicts are encouraged to help teach their clients how to more intuitively sense their body's signals of fatigue, overexertion, thirst, hunger, and muscle soreness. In a culture where the vast majority of fitness-related messages tell us to push ourselves harder and faster, it is all too easy for many of us—even non-exercise addicts—to ignore or discount our distress or discomfort. Pushing past the pain isn't always a viable option—and the exercise addict must learn to let go of this type of detrimental advice.

Support is an enormous part of recovery. Changing our default, well-practiced behaviors involves making conscious decisions to act differently or to hold ourselves back from performing those activities that we know are bad for us. Because behavioral change initially entails a period of practicing things we don't particularly like (i.e., for the exercise addict, putting a time limit on gym sessions), adherence to healthier regimens requires reinforcement from multiple angles. Having a solid network of friends, mental health professionals, and knowledgeable fitness professionals who can offer encouragement to the recovering exercise addict helps to bolster his or her circumvention of self-destructive activity patterns. (For starters, readers can take advantage of the resources listed in appendix A.) Any recovering exercise addict looking to change must understand that overcoming a well-ingrained habit won't happen overnight. However, numerous primary and secondary overexercisers have emerged from the confines of their obsessive fitness habits into happier, healthier, and more satisfying lives, proving that change is entirely possible.

Recovery occurs when the goal of physical activity shifts from the annihilation of neediness and avoidance of helplessness to the function of self-regulation and pleasure. Rarely does a person feel compelled to exercise excessively when she experiences her body as an extension of herself that is to be enjoyed and cared for rather than beaten into submission or overly controlled. A recovered exercise addict no longer feels the need to cycle through the same repetitive pattern of physical activities day in and day out, nor does she feel an overwhelming onslaught of anxiety if her exercise plans must be rearranged to make room for social, professional, or personal obligations. Although she may be frustrated when she can't work out as anticipated, she takes heart in the newly found flexibility of incorporating exercise as one part of her life rather than as its sole, relentless purpose.

9

HOW TO APPROACH SOMEONE WITH A PROBLEM

Many readers may have picked up *The Truth about Exercise Addiction* because they've witnessed a friend or loved one use exercise in a self-destructive manner. If you count yourself among this cohort, you might be considering how to confront someone you believe has a problem. As with any type of intervention, drawing attention to an exercise addict's behavior may seem intimidating. But with the right communication tools, expressing concern about someone's unhealthy habits may enable him or her to get needed help. What follows are some guidelines and tips to keep in mind when approaching a person caught in the throes of exercise addiction.

The first step in determining what to say to an exercise addict (and how to say it) involves comprehending the scope of the relationship you have with him or her. A close family member has a different emotional leverage than a romantic partner, just as a personal trainer has a different angle of experience than a fellow gym-goer or even a nonactive friend.

The closer you are to the exercise addict, the better. A strong rapport can heavily influence how likely the exercise addict is to trust or even to be open to hearing what you have to say. Keep in mind that most exercise addicts cling to working out not just as their preferred—if not sole—coping mechanism, but also as a means of confirming their identity and self-worth. As such, they are highly unlikely to be amenable to the idea that their fitness efforts are a cause for concern, and they'll

most likely be heavily resistant to the notion that their lifestyle should
be altered in some radical way. The exercise addict may not even be
able to envision an existence that fluidly incorporates pursuits apart
from the gym (or the daily jog, bike, or swim). So be sure to remain
sensitive to the rigidly narrowed mind-set characteristic of someone
who sidelines friends, family, and fun in favor of fitness. Understand
that it may take a high level of patience and persistence through multiple confrontations before the exercise addict will be able to consider his
or her exercise habits as problematic.

The more distant you are from the source of your concern, the more
you may want to consider conferring with the spouse, close friend,
trainer, or coach of an exercise addict. Given the strength of the relationship these latter individuals can be assumed to have with an overexerciser, not to mention the time they've likely spent observing his or her
deleterious behavior, they may be in a more appropriate place to confront the individual.

**If you qualify as a close or significant other to an exercise
addict**, be sure to offer tangible examples of what you see as the exercise addict's worrisome behavior. For instance, you may be able to point
out how your friend or loved one has been increasingly absent at social
gatherings, more exhausted and irritable than usual, and clearly harried.
Underscoring these observations, you might try simply couching your
concern in the question, "Why do you push yourself so hard?" or "Do
you ever take days off? Why not?"

Do not approach the exercise addict during a workout. Wait
for a moment where he or she is in a relatively calm state, preferably
after his or her regimen has been completed so that it's not at the
forefront of his or her mind, and shoot for a day you've both gotten
adequate rest. Finding a time when the exercise addict has been able to
eat something, so emotions aren't heightened by hunger, is also prefer-
able.

**Confronting an exercise addict is not an opportunity to give
advice or to itemize a list of duties he or she *should be* fulfilling
in lieu of exercise.** The very fact that you are expressing concern
about his or her habits will likely provoke enough anxiety, if not guilt
(depending on the exercise addict's awareness about how his or her
habits are affecting others).

You may also want to **avoid addiction terminology** when speaking directly to the person who you believe has a problem. Labeling can often be perceived as accusatory by those on the receiving end of even a well-meaning attempt to better identify issues, resulting in even greater resistance and emotional shutdown. Leave the diagnoses to the professionals. If the person you are confronting sounds open to your worries, encouraging him or her to consult with a mental health professional may be in order—especially if you, yourself, have experience with therapy or know someone who greatly benefitted from it. "My therapist really helped me get over that depression/bad habit/anxiety I used to struggle with" is more inviting than "I've never had to see a therapist but maybe you should." Singling out the exercise addict without demonstrating how you can, in some way (even if by a long shot), relate may serve only to further alienate him or her.

Another tip to keep in mind is to **avoid expressing amazement, bafflement, or awe at the exercise addict's behavior**. Statements like "I just don't understand why you feel the need to do all that," "Your behavior is insane," or "I can't even imagine how you exercise so much" underscore the exercise addict's otherness, heightening his or her sense of isolation and separateness from you, the concerned individual. Instead, try couching your worry in terms of understanding—"I know what it's like to feel you can't live without something"—or empathy—"I can imagine how it might be stressful and exhausting to feel like you have to run for two hours every morning before doing anything else."

Individuals with a fitness background (i.e., personal trainers) who have close contact with someone they think might be using fitness self-destructively **can use their knowledge of exercise science as an inroad to highlight the harm in an exercise addict's habits**. Pointing out the body's physiological need for rest and recovery, along with the very real physical consequences of overuse, may be the best way to communicate the necessity of scaling back to someone compelled to work out without pause. Fitness professionals who have witnessed or personally experienced an injury due to overexercising or inadequate recovery may want to share such stories as illustrations of what the exercise addict can expect if he or she does not cut back.

When staff at a fitness facility are concerned about a particular member's physical well-being, it is within their scope of practice to request medical clearance from the person about whom they are concerned. Jodi Rubin, a therapist specializing in eating disorders and over-zealous exercise habits, likens this simple procedure to the steps health club employees might take for members with a high risk of heart attack. Through Destructively Fit, a series of courses designed to educate fitness professionals about eating disorders and overexercise, Rubin works with personal trainers and exercise instructors to help them identify clients' unhealthy habits at the gym. She emphasizes that much of a fitness professional's role in confronting members' self-destructive behaviors entails compassionately expressing concern about observable shifts in their mood, energy levels, and/or behavior.

"I recommend to trainers that they lay out what they're noticing in a nonconfrontational way," explains Rubin. "It's better to phrase these observations around what you've seen change in this person rather than list all the things you think they're doing wrong." Rubin also advises fitness professionals to be patient with clients who spend too much time at the gym. "A person who overexercises is utilizing an effective yet dangerous coping mechanism. Just because you may be ready to say 'I'm worried' doesn't mean that the overexerciser is willing to admit something is going on with them. Overexercisers may insist they don't have a problem for quite a while. But by taking the risk to empathetically express your worries, you're setting the stage for future conversations. Pointing out shifts in mood and raising concerns with compassion allows a client struggling with eating or exercise issues to see you as caring, there for them, and nonjudgmental. The point is to set yourself up as someone who, when the overexerciser is ready, they feel they can talk to."

Relaying the potential consequences of too much time spent in motion may be the most effective means of getting through to an exercise addict. The possibility that such repercussions may ultimately prevent exercise addicts from engaging in their most coveted behavior may have more of an impact upon their consideration of change than hearing about who or what is suffering as a result of their relentless workout schedule. Remember that the appeal of activities other than those at the gym (think: quality time with friends, going to dinners, attending live theater performances or watching a movie, even traveling) is eclipsed in the exercise addict's mind by their compulsion to burn more calories, lift more weights, or hit the pavement for hours on end. To harp on what the exercise addict is missing may not be as influential in shifting his or her perspective as emphasizing how too much time spent in motion could ultimately prevent him or her from getting to the gym at all.

Instead of overtly chastising the exercise addict for how negatively his or her behavior has impacted other people (or his or her academic or professional performance), spouses, significant others, close family members, and friends can also **compassionately express how much the exercise addict is missed as an integral part of a social group or community**. Indicating a sense of personal loss without accusing the exercise addict of shirking yet another obligation may have a better chance of softening the exercise addict to the notion that his or her behavior is getting in the way of meaningful connections to others. "I miss you" is a very simple and honest statement that avoids the potentially off-putting charge that the exercise addict is doing something wrong. Moral sentiment is out of place during caring confrontations. Consider the difference between the following phrases: "I feel neglected and alone when you go to the gym instead of having brunch with me or when you prioritize running over relaxing with me on a vacation" versus "You never pay enough attention to me; you're too preoccupied with the gym." Which sounds more compassionate and inviting? (Answer: the former.)

As founding director of New York City's Eating Disorder Resource Center (EDRC) and coauthor of *Surviving an Eating Disorder*, Judith Brisman explains that those who are concerned about someone who is suffering from exercise addiction must wrap their minds around a seemingly counterintuitive premise: rarely is an exercise addict's behavior about exercise alone. The obsession about calories burnt, distance logged, or weights lifted (not to mention the total amount of time spent moving) fulfills a fundamental psychological need for the exercise addict. For some, the goal is to establish a sense of separateness, individuation, or confirmation of one's own value. For others, it is a means of quelling anxiety, guilt, and self-consciousness. Overzealous exercisers may also be compelled to work out as a means of purging excess calories, remaining thin, or bulking up and being strong so as to render themselves worthy of love and attention from others. In many cases, relentless physical activity fulfills all needs mentioned earlier. But because it does so contingently, its solutions to problems of low self-worth, diffuse identity, and anxiety are fleeting at best.

Brisman advises all individuals gearing up to confront someone who they believe suffers from an exercise addiction to keep it simple. To do this, she offers three suggestions:

1. **Stick to the facts.** With kindness, state what you've observed about the exercise addict's behavior (i.e., "I notice you've been running more and more lately. You used to run for about twenty to forty minutes. Now you're out for more than an hour. The other day you went running for so long that you missed the party we were planning to go to.").

2. **Discuss how the exercise addict's behavior is affecting your relationship.** Here's the opportunity to tell him or her how you feel. For instance: "I miss you. I feel like you don't want to spend any time with me. It seems like you'd rather be at the gym than sit down and have dinner with me and that hurts."

3. **Be clear (and reasonable) about what you would like the exercise addict to do.** This might mean that you ask him or her to seek professional help, to schedule one day a week away from the gym to make more time for friends and family, or to see a doctor regarding an injury. (Note: you'll want to keep these suggestions practical. No one who has been working out every day for a significant period of time will take kindly to the notion of cutting out exercise altogether. Baby steps are more palatable than 180-degree shifts.)

"To tell exercise addicts that you want them to stop exercising altogether is not reasonable," Brisman explains. "That misses the question of why they are doing it to begin with. You're really trying to reengage them back in the world. Instead of saying 'You must not exercise at all,' point to what you are concerned about and then try asking the exercise addict 'What can I give you, instead?' The point is to give them a feasible goal they can work toward."

The less accusatory you can be when pointing out an exercise addict's potential problem(s), the better. Obviously this requires a great deal of self-restraint on the part of the confronter. Those struggling to make sense of, relate to, or intervene on an exercise addict's behalf may do well to seek out a mental health professional of their own. In addition to having a trusted ally in whom they can confide their frustration, concern, and sense of relational rupture, friends and loved ones of exercise addicts may do well to examine if or how they might be contributing to an exercise addict's injurious habits. **Many of us inadvertently encourage unhealthy attitudes toward exercise** merely by endorsing a "more is always better" approach to fitness; by actively criticizing the apparent laziness or physical appearance of others; by lavishing praise upon people who prioritize strength or endurance training above most other life activities; or by endorsing air-brushed ideals of muscularity and thinness.

Brisman offers the example of families who are highly fitness oriented and place a heavy (no pun intended) emphasis on physique or avoiding laziness and sloth. In these cases parents or spouses who are concerned about a child or family member's overzealous exercise habits may need to reevaluate their entrapment in the do-as-I-say-not-as-I-do paradigm whereby they plead with the exercise addict to ease off from working out yet do not demonstrate alternative behavior patterns or offer equal praise, love, and attention for activities other than fitness.

"It's tricky," admits Brisman, "but family members especially need to ask themselves whether they're doing everything they can to guide the exercise addict toward healthier goals. That takes a lot of self-awareness."

It may also be the case that a parent or loved one is too overbearing with an exercise addict and that what really needs to happen before any progress can be made is for this ostensibly caring individual to take a few steps back. Brisman has seen many parents who assume "they just need to try harder in order for their kid to change. What they don't realize is that all the things they keep trying to do are making the situation worse."

Backing off may be difficult, especially when a child or loved one's health seems to be in danger. In the event that a person's physical well-being is at stake, more drastic measures—such as restricting access to the gym, accompanying a loved one to doctors appointments, or considering a temporary hospitalization—may be in order. (In the event a person cannot take care of him- or herself, he or she is essentially forfeiting his autonomy.)

Distancing oneself from the sufferer can be additionally complicated by the risk that ignoring an exercise addict's behavior inadvertently communicates a lack of caring.

"Ultimately, parents, family members, spouses, or friends need to attend to the fact that someone is really in trouble," explains Brisman. Allowing the exercise addict to experience some consequences of his or her behavior may be necessary for him or her to realize why he or she should ease off. But when someone's physical and emotional health is clearly being damaged, those who really care about the exercise addict must intervene.

The key to encouraging an exercise addict to reevaluate his or her relationship to fitness is to convey care and love rather than accusation or threats. "What you can do," Brisman says, "is set the stage for recovery. You have the right to say 'We're in trouble. I'm losing you. And we need to talk to someone. How can I help you come back?'"

It is the unfortunate reality of all mental illnesses and addictions that true recovery and behavioral change cannot be forced upon a sufferer regardless of how well intentioned a concerned other's insistence may be. Unless an exercise addict is hospitalized or committed to an inpatient facility, the amount he or she exercises (and the degree to which he or she refuels and rests after periods of overexertion) is an autonomous decision. Support, concern, and confrontation can only go so far.

Many friends and loved ones who know an exercise addict may not initially succeed in getting through to them. It is not uncommon for exercise addicts to persist in their overzealous habits until injury occurs, and even when their health is endangered they may remain unwilling to cut back their workouts. In cases of extreme resistance, sometimes the best thing that those who are worried about someone they love can do is to experiment with encouraging activities that do not involve excess physical exertion but rather that provide an opportunity for the exercise addict to build self-worth, have fun, feel included, or simply relax. This may be the hardest experiment of all, considering that exercise addicts may resist activities that appeal to nonaddicts because they interfere with maximizing the time spent exercising. Sneaking in such activities around workouts may be the best that caring friends and family members can do.

There does come a point, however, where healthy limits must be set in order to protect those who are expending too much of their own energy on trying to solve the exercise addict's issue. When the amount of time spent worrying or caring for the exercise addict begins to pull a caring friend or loved one away from his or her life, this is a cause for concern—and a sign of codependency. Codependency occurs frequently in cases of both behavioral and chemical addictions and also is quite common in families whose members suffer from eating disorders. While the exercise addict may predicate his self-esteem on how much he can lift or how far he can run, a codependent partner, friend, or family member may place an equal amount of importance on his or her ability to control the exercise addict's behavior or "be there" for him in times of need. Putting the exercise addict's needs before their own; being on continual alert for issues; suffering anxiety, depression, and hopelessness; and walking on eggshells are additional signs of codependency that are often reported by individuals dealing with someone who is suffering from addiction or disorder eating. That codependency often goes unnoticed by all parties involved is yet another reason individuals in close relationships with an exercise addict may do well to seek mental health support of their own.

10

FREQUENTLY ASKED QUESTIONS

Is exercise addiction another form of obsessive-compulsive disorder (OCD)?

Exercise addiction isn't just another iteration of obsessive-compulsive disorder. Although it certainly involves obsessive thinking habits and ritualistic behaviors, exercise addiction is additionally characterized by tolerance (the need to increase the time spent performing the behavior to achieve its initial euphoria-producing or anxiety-relieving effects). Unlike obsessive-compulsive disorder, exercise addiction is also characterized (at least, in its early stages) by the pursuit of pleasure via the compulsive activity, rather than just the release from (emotional or physical) pain. (Over time, the pleasure afforded by exercise diminishes and withdrawal—or, the avoidance of anxiety and guilt affiliated with missing a workout day—becomes the primary motivation to persist in the activity.)

Another factor that separates exercise addiction from obsessive-compulsive disorder is its rooting in reality. Whereas individuals suffering from behavioral compulsions are often aware of the absurdity of their urges, an exercise addict often believes the fears fueling his compulsive behavior are realistic (even if they are overblown). Common worries exercise addicts report include fear of weight gain, fear of losing muscle, fear of not working hard enough, and fear of being worthless in the absence of the effort put toward physical exertion.

What makes exercise addiction different from an eating disorder?

Although abuse of exercise is frequently a component of anorexia or bulimia nervosa, exercise addiction isn't always affiliated with a desire to lose weight, burn fat, or purge calories. Though secondary exercise addiction (i.e., compulsive exercise behavior in service of an eating disorder) may comprise the majority of cases, primary exercise addiction sufferers do exist. Bodybuilders obsessed with building muscle mass and gaining strength may qualify as primary exercise addicts, as might obligatory runners and other obsessively driven athletes who aren't as concerned with pursuing inhuman thinness as they are with pursuing physical activity as an end in itself. (The goal for primary exercise addicts may be simply to remain in motion as often as possible, continually occupied so as not to fall into a feared trap of stillness.)

Do other addictions or disorders coincide with exercise addiction?

Eating disorders are the most frequent co-occurring pathologies among exercise addicts. Some evidence suggests up to 20 percent of exercise addicts are also addicted to cigarettes, illegal substances, and alcohol.[1] Exercise addicts also may be more prone to sex addiction[2] and compulsive shopping.[3, 4] Though the professional lives of exercise addicts may be hampered as a result of the time they spend working out, a number of exercise addicts also have been shown to be prone to "work addiction."[5] Caffeine use and stimulant or steroid use is also much higher among exercise addicts, who lean on such substances to facilitate the intensity of their overzealous workouts.[6, 7]

Is being addicted to exercise really all that bad?

Though you might think exercise is the least harmful addictive behavior, the numerous physical and psychological consequences of the disorder are no insignificant matter. Physical tolls of overexercise include heart abnormalities (from arrhythmias to scarring and sudden cardiac arrest), bone fractures or breaks, muscle tears, ligament strains, hernias, dehydration and fatigue, heat exhaustion, and kidney failure. That doesn't even begin to account for long-term consequences, like a potentially reduced life expectancy due to chronic overexertion, higher susceptibility to arthritis and osteoporosis, along with temporary and prolonged infertility in women.

On the psychological level, irritability, anxiety, depression, and mood swings result not only from not taking enough off days, but also from the isolation and lost work productivity most exercise addicts experience as a consequence of too much time spent working out.

Do you have to work out for hours and hours each day to qualify as an exercise addict?

Although a major hallmark of exercise addiction is tolerance—needing more and more of the activity to achieve its initially desired results—and a noticeable amount of time spent in motion, not all exercise addicts spend hours and hours each day working out. (Some, in fact, do manage to take days off—despite feeling lethargic, short-tempered, easily agitated, and anxious until they can get back to the gym the following day.)

Exercise addiction begins when individuals steadily increase their workout times in order to chase the initial high they experienced from cardiovascular activities, strength training, or other types of physical exertion. The time someone spends working out is only one criterion of seven (see chapter 2, "What It Looks Like: The Signs and Symptoms of Exercise Addiction") that determine whether he or she qualifies as addicted. Usually, an exercise addict will spend a noticeable amount of time exerting him- or herself comparable to his or her friends and colleagues. However, if a person's previously satisfying twenty-minute run (or lifting session) begins to feel inadequate along with a reduction in time spent on other previously enjoyable activities, persistence even when sick or injured, and excessive guilt or anxiety in the face of keeping one's time spent in motion within reason, he or she may qualify as addicted. Put simply: a person who is hooked on physical activity devotes a great deal of time to exercise, but there's no precise number at which one can automatically be considered an exercise addict. Time is just one of seven factors mental health professionals must weigh when assessing whether someone is addicted to working out. Generally speaking, physical activity that continuously extends two hours or more can be considered a red flag, but even at lesser numbers a person can be suffering.

Do all exercise addicts look muscular and skinny?

A common misconception about exercise addiction is that all sufferers will be immensely toned, thin, or hypermuscular. This isn't necessarily the case. Keep in mind when you don't take time off, adequately refuel, and let your body recover from the repeated stress exercise entails, your muscles are at a higher risk of atrophying. (There's a reason personal trainers suggest that clients looking to build muscle may want to reduce their cardio and increase their protein consumption.)

Although those who pursue physical activity on a regular basis are more likely to be thinner and more sculpted than those who spend most of their time on the couch, the body's appearance has little to do with what qualifies someone as addicted to exercise. The pathology lies in the behavior surrounding working out as much as the attitude and belief system that drives that behavior. The black-and-white conclusion that *I cannot function if I don't go to the gym and burn four hundred calories before work* is distorted, regardless of what those daily burn sessions result in, physically speaking. Likewise, the need to persist in physical activity despite illness and against the advice of a medical professional is also unsound. Even if someone has lost muscle tone due to not physically being able to run, bike, swim, or lift as much, that they still feel intolerable guilt and anxiety in response to exercising less is indicative of addiction.

I feel guilty/anxious/crabby when I don't get to the gym. Am I addicted to exercise?

Not necessarily. The withdrawal symptoms of irritability, anxiety, and guilt (also depressed mood) aren't the only qualifiers of exercise addiction. Most folks who exercise regularly experience slight dips in mood when they miss a regular workout or are prevented from moving in a way that makes them feel good. If these mood dips become increasingly unbearable and prevent someone from functioning, however, that's a sign that something may be more serious. (People without an exercise addiction can tolerate the frustration of not getting to the gym and get on with the rest of their day, trusting that they can make up for lost time or simply accepting the fact that they may not be able to. The exercise addict feels emotionally debilitated in the event she misses a workout and struggles to adequately function until she gets her next "fix.")

If I exercise every day (or almost every day) am I addicted to exercise?

Some people who go to the gym every day are irrefutably addicted. Others appear to be free of addiction, considering they make time for other activities and aren't obsessive about their routines. Whether you are addicted to exercise depends on how your daily (or near daily) workouts affect your mental and physical health, your social life, and your ability to function in non-exercise-related endeavors. If you find yourself constantly exhausted, intolerably anxious at the thought of missing a workout, or unable to muster enough energy for activities that don't involve burning calories or lifting weights, you may have a problem. To be considered addicted to exercise a person must fulfill at least three or more criteria from the Exercise Dependence Scale in appendix B.

Are athletes addicted to exercise?

The rates of exercise addiction among athletes are, as you might expect, much higher than in the general population. Only 3 percent of the general public is thought to suffer from exercise addiction while 25 percent of runners[8] qualify as addicted to their sport. Take a look at triathletes and that percentage burgeons to 52 percent.[9] Among a random sample of regular gym-goers, that number sprang to 42 percent in one study.[10] Intriguingly, 7 percent of sports science majors at the college or graduate level meet the criteria for exercise addiction.[11, 12]

Among nonprofessional athletes and regular exercisers whose sport of choice emphasizes thinness or muscularity (i.e., dancing or bodybuilding), disturbances in self-perception and remarkable discomfort with one's body are far higher than in the general population.[13]

That said, just because an individual engages in a sport for competitive or leisure purposes does not mean he or she automatically qualifies for exercise addiction. In fact, someone could spend up to an hour or two a day in motion and still not be considered an exercise addict. Addiction creeps in when the pursuit of the sport or the engagement in physical activity takes precedence over all else in that person's life. Even athletes take off days, go out with friends, fulfill their roles as parents, significant others, or (if they're at the professional level) publicity demands. If an athlete repeatedly feels compelled to practice beyond the recommendations of his or her coach or trainer, that's a red flag. If he or she continually obsesses about getting in a morning run before the afternoon track meet or finishing up at a gym if a race or a game doesn't feel like *enough*, that's another red flag.

How does body image relate to exercise addiction?

Individuals who fit the bill for primary exercise addiction (read: those who crave constant motion rather than calorie burning or muscle building) may not suffer from body image issues. For those who qualify as secondary exercise addicts, however, poor body image may be a strong contributor to their pathology.

These individuals' low self-image may fuel the desire to continually work toward burning more calories or increasing muscle tone so as to make themselves look (and feel) more acceptable. Secondary exercise addicts with impaired body image feel compelled to exercise ad nauseam, tirelessly trying to keep their contingent self-esteem afloat via how much they can accomplish by working out. To the exercise addict, breaks from physical activity mean not only physical lethargy and irritability, but the crash of a self-worth predicated primarily on fitness accomplishments.

Are some exercises more addictive than others?

Running (and other high-intensity cardiovascular activities, like cycling, swimming, or intense elliptical or Stairmaster sessions) tend to elicit endorphins more strongly, but an exercise addict can easily latch onto any type of repetitive exertion to fuel his or her addiction. The answer to this question is complicated by the fact that many studies on exercise addiction focus on aerobic training more often than, say, strength training, yoga, or Pilates. There is currently no data confirming whether one type of exercise is more addictive than another. An exercise addict's preferred routine depends in large part on what is available to him or her, what he or she has learned to master, and what purpose (i.e., burning calories, increasing muscle mass, or simply remaining in motion) his or her chosen exercise serves.

Who is more likely to become addicted to exercise: men or women?

According to several studies, men appear to report more exercise addiction symptoms than women.[14, 15, 16] One explanation for this disparity boils down to each gender's means of pursuing their desired physique: Men may take more readily to exercise as it promises to confer a more muscular appearance in line with stereotypical male standards of beauty. Women, on the other hand, may be more inclined to use diet in striving toward their stereotypical female standards of beauty (namely, thinness).[17]

That said, women tend to be at a higher risk of eating disorders than men. And approximately half of all eating disorders are thought to involve exercise as a means to curtail weight gain or to purge excess calories. When exercise is used as a means to achieve or maintain an unhealthily low weight, it is all the more dangerous. Malnutrition coupled with exercise markedly raises the physical consequences of pathological physical activity levels, predisposing eating-disordered overexercisers to organ damage, abnormalities in (or loss of) hair, skin, and bone density (teeth included), and menstrual irregularities, including temporary and prolonged infertility. Incidence of exercise addiction may be lower among women, but the severity of their symptoms is comparable to the severity of men's—if not further exacerbated by accompanying eating-disordered behavior.

Are certain personality traits predictive of developing exercise addiction?

Although personality isn't the *only* factor contributing to a person's likelihood of becoming addicted to exercise, research has demonstrated a higher prevalence of exercise addiction symptoms among extraverts, perfectionists, those scoring high on neuroticism, and people who display lower levels of agreeability. Psychologists believe the stamina required to maintain an addiction to exercise can feed off a typical extravert's high energy levels, while perfectionism and neuroticism often lead to compulsive behaviors.[18] Low levels of agreeability are linked with competitiveness and egocentrism.

By contrast, friendliness, emotional stability, and conscientiousness appear to insulate individuals from the risk of developing exercise addiction, as these qualities tend to render people more behaviorally flexible, socially connected, and self-aware in a manner that promotes controlling impulses and exercising in moderation.

If you work out multiple hours a day for most days of the week without getting hurt or missing much socialization are you an addict?

It's not just about how long you work out. Certainly, you can be an incredibly active person and still make time for family, work, and fun. That said, there's evidence that working out for more than two-and-a-half hours each day is indicative of a less healthy drive that may ultimately undermine well-being.[19] Heath benefits of daily exercise seem to max out between forty-five minutes (if the exercise is vigorous) and 110 minutes (if the exercise is light to moderate).[20] To push beyond this may indicate a desire for something unrelated to health—perhaps a competitive edge that leads one to injury or a desire to tirelessly lift self-esteem that's become contingent on one's cardiovascular or strength-training output.

Frequency is not the only component of addiction. Tolerance, withdrawal, intention effect, and persistence in spite of injury or illness also factor into what qualifies someone as an exercise addict. If the person exercising for multiple hours a day yet still making time for family and friends continues to work out before social events, despite an injury, or plans to go to the gym in the morning for only forty-five minutes but finds himself staying for an hour and a half and getting to work just in the nick of time, these may be red flags that indicate his passion is verging on pathology. If the reason he works out so many hours a day is to offset the guilt and anxiety associated with not completing a compulsive routine even while fulfilling many other obligations in his life, this is also problematic.

Exercise addiction isn't black and white. Its severity comes in degrees. The more criteria an individual meets on the Exercise Dependence Scale, the more deeply enmeshed she is in her addiction.

Does exercise addiction decrease with age?

Yes. Research shows that symptoms of exercise addiction decrease with age, typically hitting their lowest levels after age forty-five.[21] Eighteen to twenty-four-year-olds seem to be at the highest risk for exercise addiction, with twenty-five to forty-four-year-olds trailing closely behind. Researchers surmise this is due in part to the inevitable reduction in physical activity that comes with aging along with older adults' better-honed abilities to regulate their emotions.[22, 23]

Is it okay for exercise addicts to have workout equipment in their own home?

Many exercise addicts may be triggered by having workout equipment in their homes. If they live alone, the risk of relapse may be heightened, as others aren't around to interfere with—or monitor—potential resumptions of unhealthy behavior. This isn't to say that exercise addicts (or those who've suffered symptoms in the past) should give up physical activity in the home. But keeping cardiovascular machines or weights close at hand could reinforce the exercise addict's sense of obligation to use the equipment, along with perpetuating the exercise addict's focus on physical activity despite a range of other enjoyable and healthy alternatives.

An exercise addict looking to realize a healthier relationship to physical activity should speak with their individual treatment providers to map out what a reasonable use of at-home equipment entails. If the exercise addict is at a point in his or her life where she or he can utilize the equipment without exceeding limits (established with a trainer sensitive to exercise addiction or with a mental health professional), having equipment at home can be manageable.

Is it bad to invite exercise addicts to partake in physically exerting activities? (If someone I know suffers from exercise addiction, should I avoid inviting her to a spin class or asking her to go jogging with me?)

It depends on the severity of the exercise addict's symptoms, whether or not the activity you participate in with him or her will be substituted for or added on to his or her daily routine, and whether you are concerned for the exercise addict's physical and emotional health. If an exercise addict is below a healthy weight, injured, ill, or has recently expressed anxiety about working out to you, it may be best to avoid suggesting a physically exerting outing. Instead, try inviting him or her to a meditation class or for a leisurely walk. It is also important to consider what other exercise he or she has done that day or during the past few days. Instead of encouraging him or her to repeat the same exercise, it is best to encourage variation.

The tricky thing here is that exercise itself isn't bad. Nor should someone who identifies with the symptoms of exercise addiction assume that all forms of physical activity will be sources of self-abuse. If the exercise addict is learning how to integrate working out into his or her life more moderately, it may indeed help to exercise with a friend who understands moderation and who does not struggle with symptoms of exercise addiction (or an eating disorder). A common consequence of exercise addiction is that it drives the sufferer into isolation. Many exercise addicts avoid working out with others—or if they run, lift, or swim with a pal, they fixate on competitively inching ahead of their pals. It may be beneficial for exercise addicts to see a close friend model a healthy relationship with exercise. In this case, encouraging a friend who suffers from overzealous exertion to engage in an activity you both can do moderately may be helpful to his or her recovery.

Your best bet is to be sensitive to the exercise addict's anxiety surrounding the activity and to be able to sniff out signs he or she is pushing him- or herself too hard. Try extending a nonjudgmental ear to your friend by inviting him or her to share feelings and thoughts related to exercise as you both go about it. Reassure him or her that you're there for support, not as an unwelcome challenge!

What are the signs that someone is an exercise addict?

Most significantly: exercise dominates the person's life. They spend more and more time at the gym. They cancel plans with friends or family to sneak in gym sessions. They need more and more time in motion to achieve the initial effects of calmness, reduced guilt, or euphoria that exercise initially provided. Nervousness when not active may be a sign. And the kicker: exercising despite illness or injury.

Is an exercise addict capable of making rational decisions regarding physical activity?

The core of addiction is a loss of control over self-control in the face of a behavior or substance. With this loss of control comes a loosened grip on rationality. Whether or not an exercise addict can be trusted to make sound decisions regarding the amount of activity in which he or she can reasonably engage is debated by mental health professionals and grows increasingly thornier when we recall that compulsion often eclipses will. When it comes to pursuing moderation in physical activity and approaching exercise in a balanced, non-excessive manner, exercise addicts may be incapable of understanding how much (i.e., how long or how intensely) they really should be working out. Many exercise addicts have conditioned themselves to ignore their body's fatigue and distress signals to an extent that they are truly incapable of intuitively knowing when to stop. That they have repeatedly practiced (read: reinforced) their chosen exercise habits for months, if not years or sometimes decades, has rendered working out not just a default, automatic behavior, but also a seemingly sole coping mechanism for just about every life stressor—despite the immense amount of physical, social, and psychological stress the exercise behavior adds to an exercise addict's life. Thinking outside the exercise bubble is, therefore, incredibly difficult for the exercise addict. Factoring in consequences, alternative coping strategies, and a reasonable consideration of bodily and emotional needs thus may be challenging for an exercise addict, who must relearn acceptable and reasonable amounts of physical activity. Until he or she has deciphered with a therapist, fitness professional, or medical professional what a reasonable amount of exercise entails, the argument can be made that the exercise addict is temporarily incapable of understanding where to draw the line in terms of working out.

Are there environmental factors that contribute to exercise addiction?

Our culture is steeped in slogans disregarding moderation in physical activity. We're tirelessly pushed to work harder, run faster, and be stronger—in *and* out of the gym. These social messages feed the exercise addicts' mind-set, and perpetuate an unquestioned blanket approval of any and all time spent at the gym.

Fitness marketing and media also fuel the individualistic, competitive pursuit of physical perfection toward which the exercise addict continually toils. Although motivational messages surrounding exercise may help some folks sustain reasonable physical activity levels, they can be detrimental to exercise addicts by providing justifications for unhealthy levels of exercise. Such messages can also amplify the exercise addict's guilt for not living up to inhumanly in-shape standards.

What is the fitness professional's role in identifying and treating exercise addiction?

Personal trainers, gym managers, and fitness instructors are not mental health professionals. For them to attempt to "treat" the pathology of exercise addiction is beyond their scope of practice. Employees in the fitness industry are, however, often in a prime position to detect exercise addiction symptoms. If a personal trainer or instructor has a close relationship with a gym-goer that he or she believes may have a problem, it may be reasonable for him or her to approach that person. (For tips on approaching exercise addicts, please refer to chapter 9.) The knowledge base possessed by those who are trained and certified in exercise physiology can be a valuable tool in conveying to exercise addicts the importance of slowing down, the dangers inherent in overtraining, and the necessity of moderation.

Like most folks who are not aware of the signs and symptoms of exercise addiction, many fitness professionals can all too easily fall into the trap of inadvertently encouraging unhealthy habits at the gym simply by offering undiscriminating praise and approval for all exercise-related feats. Slogans like "no pain, no gain" or the validating "congratulations!" offered to exercise addicts who increase the speed, intensity, or frequency of their workouts despite detriments to health may unintentionally reinforce a nonstop attitude that risks undermining well-being in the long run and shutting down the self-awareness that enables moderation.

Is exercise addiction inherited, like alcoholism?

The genetic risk factors that render people vulnerable for substance addictions may put them at equal risk for behavioral addictions, like exercise addiction.[24] Rats, for instance, who display high preferences for addictive drugs also display equally high preferences for staying glued to their running wheels. Many humans who discontinue their excessive drug or alcohol use may also be more susceptible to drug or alcohol abuse—as well as other addictions. There may indeed be an addictive personality profile, compounded by an individual's early life experiences, that sets him or her up for addiction. Much of this may boil down to a hyperactive dopamine system in the reward centers of the brain. Whether he falls in with a crowd where drugs offer him that sense of *just being okay* or whether he takes up physical activity to offset feelings of low self-esteem and to get his proverbial fix may be a function of what he has at his disposal when he's learning how to cope with life's stressors.

Lending credence to the notion that exercise addicts' brains may simply be more predisposed to addictive behavior, studies show those who regularly overdo it at the gym are nearly twice as prone toward compulsive shopping than those who can keep their workouts within reason.[25]

Are there support groups for this, or is the treatment individualized?

Currently there are no support groups for exercise addiction comparable to substance abuse and behavioral addiction support. Many eating-disorder treatment centers offer counseling for overexercisers, as exercise addiction is often a component of eating-disordered behavior. Most treatments are cognitive, behavioral based, and individualized.

What are the signs of relapse?

An exercise addict can be said to be slipping back into unhealthy behavior when he or she begins to meet more criteria on the Exercise Dependence Scale: withdrawing from social or work activities (and social roles), spending increasing amounts of time at the gym, exercising despite injury or illness, and growing agitated and anxious in the event a workout is missed.

What is the life expectancy of an exercise addict?[26]

Exercising too much for too long may heighten the risk of death as much as never being physically active at all. Whereas folks who run a total of five to twenty miles per week may see their longevity increased by 25 percent, those who run more than twenty miles per week may actually decrease their longevity to levels seen in people who spend most of their lives sedentary.

What injuries do exercise addicts run the risk of incurring?

Exercise addicts are at great risk for a range of skeletal and muscular injuries from sprains (ligament tears) and strains (muscle tears) to bone spurs, stress fractures, and breaks. Over the long term, exercise addicts are more likely to develop arthritis than moderately to occasionally active individuals. If malnutrition plays into an exercise addict's compulsive physical activity habits, risks for osteoporosis (especially among women) are significantly raised. At the disorder's most severe levels, the internal organs can take heavy hits—including the kidneys, the reproductive system, and, most of all, the heart. The most extreme cases of exercise addiction run the risk of kidney failure,[27] sudden cardiac arrest,[28] and stroke.[29]

But I thought exercise was supposed to be good for your heart!

Exercising intensely for more than an hour puts significant stress on the heart, resulting in overstretching its valves and mini tears in the muscles surrounding the heart. This is a relatively normal response to exercise and contributes to strengthening the heart if the exerciser takes adequate time off from his or her workouts to recover. If the heart is not given enough time to recalibrate and recover (like the other muscles of the body), it is at a higher risk of short- and long-term injury.

Upon autopsy, the heart tissues of long-term endurance athletes exhibit inflammation, enlargement, thickening and stiffening of artery walls, and scarring. Increased incidences of arrhythmias (like atrial and ventricular fibrillation—irregular heartbeats) have been documented in veteran extreme athletes. Marathoners have a threefold increased incidence of fibrosis (an excess agglomeration of fibrous tissue) inside the walls of their heart chambers and a 60 percent increase in the accumulation of plaque within their arteries when compared to nonrunners.

In a study of patients suffering from coronary heart disease, sixty minutes of vigorous exercise worsened the stiffness of their blood vessels and increased the free radicals floating through their bloodstream, while thirty minutes of vigorous exercise improved their blood vessels' elasticity and lowered free radical levels.

If malnutrition accompanies chronic physical overexertion, the heart is subjected to even greater stress, typically atrophying in the face of inadequate fuel.

Is there a link between childhood abuse and exercise addiction?

Although some evidence exists to affirm a link between childhood abuse and eating disorders, there are (as of the publication of this book) no known studies linking exercise addiction to childhood abuse. There are, however, numerous studies linking early childhood abuse with susceptibility to addiction in adulthood,[30] along with research confirming a link between early life maltreatment and low self-esteem, a major contributing factor to many exercise addicts' unhealthy behavior. Childhood abuse has also been shown to greatly exacerbate (and potentially cause) adult anxiety, depression,[31] and neuroticism[32]—three additional factors that may play into an exercise addict's symptoms. Though not all exercise addicts should be assumed to have a history of abuse, psychological and physical violence (or neglect) could potentially contribute to exercise addiction symptoms via the former's toll on self-esteem and mood and contribution to personality factors known to give rise to pathological physical activity pursuits.

What does "recovery" from exercise addiction entail?

By no means are exercise addicts expected to forgo gyms entirely or rule out physical activity for the rest of their lives. Recovery from exercise addiction does not follow an abstinence-only model. (To pursue this route might be equally unhealthy, considering the high rates of disease associated with not exercising enough.) Rather, kicking the unhealthy habit of overzealous exercise involves mastering the fine art of flexibility and moderation in behavior.

This means sticking to a limit on exercise by creating an exercise plan with a knowledgeable trainer, physician, or mental health professional that enables exercise addicts to welcome healthy levels of activity into their lives without taking it too far.

One place to start is simply by changing the types of workouts on which exercise addicts have become so hooked. If running has become compulsive and obligatory, the exercise addict might try switching to cycling, cardio sessions on the elliptical or Stairmaster, or swimming. Strength training can also be introduced to individuals who cling to cardio as their sole means of getting a bit too much of that endorphin-rush fix. For bodybuilders looking to ease up on their weight lifting, the opposite would hold—cardio and cross-training might be better suited to help them learn new patterns of activity. Yoga and Pilates can help many exercise addicts develop a greater body awareness while focusing (and calming) the mind.

Many exercise addiction treatment professionals recommend a period of abstinence from exercise to recalibrate the body and to allow the deeper issues fueling an addictive relationship to the gym to bubble to the surface. When an exercise addict's weight has dropped to a medically unsound level, physicians recommend postponing exercise until that weight reaches a viable level. This is frequently the result of compulsive running and excess cardiovascular exertion.

The ultimate goal of getting over exercise addiction is unhinging one's self-worth from working out, finding time for other activities outside the gym, and accepting that not every day can include a two-hour training session without cycling through waves of panic and anxiety.

The true work of recovering from exercise addiction entails not just learning to limit one's self and to apply the body to endeavors apart from working out. It also involves working with a mental health professional to identify and process the emotional issues underlying why the exercise addict latched onto overzealous physical activity in the first place.

APPENDIX A: HOW TO GET HELP

Where to Go, What to Read, and to Whom to Reach Out

Resources for exercise addicts, fitness professionals, mental health specialists—and the rest of us.

BOOKS

Andersen, Arnold E., Leigh Cohn, Thomas Holbrook. *Making Weight: Men's Conflicts with Food, Weight Shape, & Appearance*. Carlsbad, CA: Gürze Books, 2000.

Andersen, Charlotte Hilton. *The Great Fitness Experiment*. Cincinatti, OH: Clerisy Press, 2011.

Arnold, Carrie. *Running on Empty: A Diary of Anorexia and Recovery*. Livonia, MI: First Page Publications, 2004.

Cash, Thomas E. *The Body Image Workbook: An Eight-Step Program for Learning to Like Your Looks*. 2nd ed. Oakland, CA: New Harbinger Publications, 1997.

Freimuth, Marilyn. *Addicted? Recognizing Destructive Behaviors before It's Too Late*. Lanham, MD: Rowman & Littlefield Publishers, 2008.

———. *Hidden Addictions: Assessment Practices for Psychotherapists, Counselors, and Health Care Providers*. Lanham, MD: Jason Aronson, 2005.

Friedman, Peach. *Diary of an Exercise Addict*. Guildford, CT: GPP Life, 2009.

Grogan, Sarah. *Body Image: Understanding Body Dissatisfaction in Men, Women and Children*. New York: Taylor & Francis, 2007.

Hussa, Robyn. *Healthy Selfitude: A Practical Approach to Self-acceptance Using Performing Arts and Yoga*. New York: White Elephant Enterprises, 2012.

Johnson, Marlys. *Understanding Exercise Addiction*. New York: Rosen Publishing Group, 2000.

Kaminker, Laura. *Exercise Addiction: When Fitness Becomes an Obsession*. New York: Rosen Publishing Group, 1998.

Kerr, John, Koenraad J. Lindner, and Michelle Blaydon. *Exercise Dependence*. New York: Routledge, 2007.

Maclean, Marion. *Defeating Anorexia Athletics: One Woman's Journey through Exercise Addiction and Beyond*. Queensland, Australia: Zeus Publications, 2010.

Morgan, John F. *The Invisible Man: A Self-help Guide for Men with Eating Disorders, Compulsive Exercise and Bigorexia*. New York: Routledge, 2008.

Paterson, Anna. *Fit to Die: Men and Eating Disorders*. Thousand Oaks, CA: Lucky Duck Books/Sage, 2004.

Phillips, Katharine. *The Broken Mirror: Understanding and Treating Body Dysmorphic Disorder*. Rev. and exp. ed. Oxford: Oxford University Press, 2005.

Pope, Harrison G., Katharine A. Phillips, and Roberto Olivardia. *The Adonis Complex: How to Identify, Treat, and Prevent Body Obsession in Men and Boys*. New York: Touchstone, 2002.

Powers, Pauline, and Ron Thompson. *The Exercise Balance*. Carlsbad, CA: Gürze Books, 2008.

Prussin, Rebecca, Philip D. Harvey, and Theresa Foy DiGeronimo. *Hooked on Exercise: How to Understand and Manage Exercise Addiction*. New York: Simon & Schuster, 1992.

Rosenberg, Kenneth Paul, and Laura Curtiss Feder. *Behavioral Addictions: Criteria, Evidence, and Treatment*. London: Elsevier, 2014.

Siegel, Michele, Judith Brisman, and Margot Weinshel. *Surviving an Eating Disorder*. New York: HarperCollins, 1997.

Sun, An-Pyng, Larry L. Ashley, and Lesley Dickson. *Behavioral Addiction: Screening, Assessment, and Treatment*. Las Vegas, NV: Central Recovery Press, 2012.

Thompson, J. Kevin, and Guy Cafri. *The Muscular Ideal: Psychological, Social, and Medical Perspectives*. Washington, DC: American Psychological Association, 2007.

Wilhelm, Sabine. *Feeling Good about the Way You Look: A Program for Overcoming Body Image Problems*. New York: Guilford Press, 2006.

Willett, Edward. *Frequently Asked Questions about Exercise Addiction*. New York: Rosen Publishing Group, 2009.

Yates, Alayne. *Compulsive Exercise and the Eating Disorders*. New York: Brunner/Mazel, 1991.

IN THE MEDIA

Allen, Arthur. "Exercise Addiction in Men." WebMD. http:// webmd.com/men/features/exercise-addiction.

Arnold, Carrie. "Exercising My Demons." *TheFix*. October 11, 2012. www.thefix.com/content/exercise-addiction-11092?page=all.

Ashton, Jennifer. "Addicted to Exercise." CBS News. November 2, 2009. www.cbsnews.com/videos/addicted-to-exercise.

Bayer, Jeff. "Training Addiction." Askmen.com. www.askmen.com/sports/bodybuilding_150/162_fitness_tip.html.

Cassata, Cathy. "Biggest Loser or Biggest Addict?" *TheFix*. March 25, 2014. www.thefix.com/content/biggest-loser-or-biggest-addict.

Clench, Sam. "Exercise Addiction: Ben Carter Tells How an Obsession with Exercise Threatened His Health." News.com.au. December 5, 2013. www.news.com.au/lifestyle/health/exercise-addiction-ben-carter-tells-how-an-obsession-with-exercise-threatened-his-health/story-fneuzlbd-1226775942243.

Cox, Lauren. "Exercise Addicts Can Blame Their Brains." ABC News. August 28, 2009. http://abcnews.go.com/Health/MensHealthNews/story?id=8430744.

Doyle, Jessica Ryen. "Woman Battles Exercise Addiction for Nearly 20 Years." Fox News. October 12, 2012. www.foxnews.com/health/2012/10/12/woman-battles-exercise-addiction-for-nearly-20-years.

"Exercise Overload: Are We Pushing Ourselves Too Far?" *Nightline*, January 16, 2014. http://abcnews.go.com/Nightline/video/exercise-overload-pushing-21552647.

Hicks, Jennifer. *Running Out*. http://vimeo.com/56173887.

Hicks, Sarah. "I'm Addicted to Exercise." Stuff.co.nz. March 27, 2014. www.stuff.co.nz/lifestyle/wellbeing/9873699/I-m-addicted-to-exercise.

Hieber, Nancy, and Michael E. Berrett, "Intuitive Exercise." *Hope & Healing* 8, no. 3 (2003): 7–9. http://centerforchange.com/news-resources/newsletter/intuitive-exercise.

Juntti, Melaina. "Are You Addicted to Exercise?" *Men's Journal*. March 19, 2014. www.mensjournal.com/health-fitness/exercise/are-you-addicted-to-exercise-20140319.

Kennard, Jerry. "Bigorexia." About.com: Men's Health. March 22, 2010. http://menshealth.about.com/cs/menonly/a/bigorexia.htm.

Lombardi, Jennifer. "Running on Empty: Exercise Compulsion and Eating Disorders." Eating Recovery Center Foundation. www.eatingrecoverycenter.com/running-on-empty.

Schreiber, Katherine. "Passion or Problem? When Exercise Becomes an Addiction." Greatist.com. June 28, 2013. http://greatist.com/fitness/exercise-addiction.

———. "I'm Legitimately Addicted to the Gym, and It's Not Pretty." xoJane.com. July 7, 2013. www.xojane.com/it-happened-to-me/addicted-to-the-gym.

Stubblefield, Heaven. "Exercise Addiction." Healthline. October 15, 2013. www.healthline.com/health/exercise-addiction?toptoctest=expand.

Tejeda, Valerie. "Eight Hours a Day of Celebrity Workouts." *TheFix*. October 24, 2012. www.thefix.com/content/exercise-addict-celebrity-workouts90811.

Woolman, Shiloh. "How Much Exercise Is Too Much?" 40/29tv.com. March 20, 2012. www.4029tv.com/How-much-exercise-is-too-much/9623504.

BLOGS

Adios Barbie: www.adiosbarbie.com
Exchanges, blog of the UNC Center of Excellence for Eating Disorders: http://uncexchanges.org
Finding Our Hunger: http://findingourhunger.com
The Great Fitness Experiment: www.thegreatfitnessexperiment.com
In My Skinny Genes: http://inmyskinnygenes.com
The Kirsten Haglund Foundation Blog: http://kirstenhaglund.com/news-blog
Monte Nido Blog: www.montenido.com/blog
Operation Beautiful: www.operationbeautiful.com
Timberline Knolls Blog: http://blog.timberlineknolls.com
We Are the Real Deal: http://wearetherealdeal.com

WEBSITES

Academy for Eating Disorders (AED): www.aedweb.org
BDD Central: www.bddcentral.com
The Body Positive: http://thebodypositive.org
Center for Change: http://centerforchange.com
Eating Disorder Activist Network: www.edactivistnetwork.org
Eating Disorders Coalition for Research, Policy, and Action (EDIC): www.eatingdisorderscoalition.org
Fuel Aotearoa: http://fuelaotearoa.co.nz
International Association of Eating Disorders Professionals Foundation: www.iaedp.com
Mental Fitness: www.normal-life.org
Multi-service Eating Disorders Association (MEDA): http://medainc.org

National Association for Males with Eating Disorders (N.A.M.E.D.): http://namedinc.org
National Eating Disoorders Association (NEDA): www.nationaleatingdisorders.org
Renfrew: www.renfrew.org
Something Fishy: www.something-fishy.org

INPATIENT AND RESIDENTIAL PROGRAMS

The following inpatient and residential facilities address exercise addiction, exercise bulimia, and/or compulsive physical activity in their treatment programs and help sufferers reprogram their relationship with fitness toward healthier goals.

- **Anna Westin Houses (The Emily Program, St. Paul, Minnesota)**

  Men, women, and adolescents
  www.emilyprogram.com/our-programs/awh
  (651) 645-5323

- **Arabella House/Linden Oaks (Naperville, Illinois)**

  Women and girls (16 and older)
  www.edward.org/workfiles/Arabellahouse.pdf
  www.edward.org/body.cfm?id=641&WT.mc_id=arabella
  (630) 355-3813

- **Avalon Hills (Logan, Utah)**

  Women and adolescent girls
  www.avalonhills.org
  (800) 330-0490
  (435) 938-6060

- **Carolina House (Durham and Raleigh, North Carolina)**

  Women only
  http://carolinahouse.crchealth.com
  (866) 690-7240

- **Castlewood (St. Louis, Missouri)**

  www.castlewoodtc.com
  (877) 628-1205

- **The Center (Edmunds, Washington)**

  Men, women, and adolescents
  www.aplaceofhope.com/eating-disorders-treatment.html
  (888) 771-5166

- **Center for Hope of the Sierras (Reno, Nevada)**

  Women and adolescent girls (16 and older)
  http://centerforhopeofthesierras.crchealth.com
  (866) 690-7242

- **Eating Recovery Center (Denver, Colorado)**

  Men and women
  www.eatingrecoverycenter.com/eating-disorder-treatment/adult-
      eating-disorders/inpatient-program
  (877) 825-8584

- **Insight Behavioral Health Centers (Northbrook, Oakbrook, Evanston, and Chicago, Illinois)**

  Men, women, and adolescents
  www.insightbhc.com
  (312) 540-9955

- **La Ventana (Thousand Oaks, California)**

  Men and women
  www.laventanaed.com
  www.laventanaed.com/about/locations/la-ventana-thousand-oaks
  (800) 560-8518

- **McCallum Place (St. Louis, Missouri)**

  Women and men
  http://www.mccallumplace.com/24-hour-residential.html
  www.mccallumplace.com/male_residential.html

(314) 968-1900

- **Mirasol**

  Women and adolescent girls
  www.mirasol.net
  www.mirasol.net/treatment-programs/residential.php
  www.mirasol.net/treatment-programs/mirasol-teen.php
  See also www.mirasol.net/treatment-programs/residential/
      healthy-exercise.php
  (888) 520-1700

- **Monte Nido (multiple locations)**

  Women only
  www.montenido.com
  (310) 457-9958
  Malibu, California: www.montenido.com/monte_nido_malibu
  Agoura Hills, California: www.montenido.com/monte_nido_vista
  Eugene, Oregon: www.rainrock.org
  Medford, Massachusetts: www.montenido.com/laurel_hill_inn

- **Montecatini (Carslbad, California)**

  Women only
  http://montecatini.crchealth.com
  (866) 762-3753

- **The Moore Center (Bellevue, Washington)**

  Women, men, adolescents, adults
  http://moorecenterclinic.com
  (425) 451-1134

- **New Dawn Treatment Center (Sausalito, California)**

  Men and women
  www.newdawntreatmentcenters.com
  (866) 969-4300

- **Oliver-Pyatt Centers (South Miami, Florida)**

  Women only

www.oliverpyattcenters.com
(866) 511-4325

- **Rader Programs (Oxnard, California)**

  Men, women, and adolescents
  www.raderprograms.com/treatment/eating-disorder-program.
     html
  www.raderprograms.com/treatment/exercise-therapy.html
  (800) 841-1515

- **Remuda Ranch (Wickenburg, Arizona)**

  Women and adolescent girls
  www.remudaranch.com
  (866) 390-5100

- **Renfrew (multiple locations)**

  Women only
  http://renfrewcenter.com
  (800) 736-3739
  Philadelphia, Pennsylvania: http://renfrewcenter.com/locations/
     residential/philadelphia-pa
  Coconut Creek, Florida: http://renfrewcenter.com/locations/
     residential/coconut-creek-fl

- **Rogers Memorial Hospital (Oconomowoc, Wisconsin)**

  Men, women, and adolescents
  http://rogershospital.org
  http://rogershospital.org/treatment-service/eating-disorders-adult-
     inpatient
  http://rogershospital.org/treatment-service/child-and-adolescent-
     inpatient-hospitalization-eating-disorders
  (800) 767-4411

- **Shoreline Center for Eating Disorder Treatment (Long Beach
  and Orange County, California)**

  Men and women
  http://shoreline-eatingdisorders.com

(562) 434-6007

- **Sierra Tucson (Tucson, Arizona)**

  Men and women
  http://sierratucson.crchealth.com/treatment/eating-disorder
  (855) 373-7752

- **Tapestry (Brevard, North Carolina)**

  Women only
  http://www.tapestrync.com/programs/residential-care.html
  (855) 396-2604

- **Timberline Knolls (Lemont, Illinois)**

  Women only
  www.timberlineknolls.com
  (855) 870-3216

- **UNC Center of Excellence for Eating Disorders (Chapel Hill, North Carolina)**

  Men and women
  www.med.unc.edu/psych/eatingdisorders/patient-care-1/
      inpatient-program
  (919) 966-7012

- **Veritas Collaborative (Durham, North Carolina)**

  Adolescents (12–19) and children (10–12)
  http://veritascollaborative.com
  (919) 908-9740

- **The Victory Program at McCallum Place (St. Louis, Missouri)**

  Specifically targeted treatments for male and female athletes
  http://thevictoryprogram.com
  (314) 968-1900

OUTPATIENT AND PARTIAL HOSPITALIZATION PROGRAMS

- **Can't Tell Network (Boca Raton, Florida)**

    Men, women, adolescents, and children
    http://canttellnetwork.com
    (888) 684-3618

- **Carolina House (Durham and Raleigh, North Carolina)**

    Women only
    http://carolinahouse.crchealth.com/
    (866) 690-7240

- **Cedar Springs (Austin, Texas)**

    Men, women, and adolescents
    http://cedarspringsaustin.com
    (800) 828-8158

- **The Center (Edmunds, Washington)**

    Men, women, and adolescents
    www.aplaceofhope.com/eating-disorders-treatment.html
    (888) 771-5166

- **Center for Hope of the Sierras (Reno, Nevada)**

    Men, women, and adolescents
    http://centerforhopeofthesierras.crchealth.com
    (866) 690-7242

- **Eating Disorder Center (Denver, Colorado)**

    Specifically targeted treatment plans for male and female athletes
    www.edcdenver.com/levels-of-care/elite-athlete-program
    (303) 771-0861

- **Eating Disorder Center of San Diego (San Diego, California)**

    Men, women, and adolescents
    http://healingwithinreach.com/adult-group-services

http://healingwithinreach.com/teen-intensive-outpatient
(858) 353-5378

- **Eating Disorder Resource Center (New York, New York)**

    www.edrcnyc.com/eating-disorder-resource-center-nyc.php
    (212) 989-3987

- **Eating Recovery Center (Denver, Colorado)**

    Men, women, adolescents, and children
    www.eatingrecoverycenter.com/eating-disorder-treatment/adult-
        eating-disorders/outpatient-services
    (877) 825-8584

- **The Emily Program (multiple locations)**

    Men, women, and adolescents
    http://www.emilyprogram.com/our-programs/outpatient_services
    (888) 364-5977

    - Seattle, Washington

        www.emilyprogram.com/locations/seattle-wa-eating-
            disorder-treatment
        (206) 283-2220

    - Spokane, Washington

        www.emilyprogram.com/locations/seattle-wa-eating-
            disorder-treatment
        (509) 252-1366

    - Duluth, Minnesota

        www.emilyprogram.com/locations/duluth-mn-eating-
            disorder-treatment
        (218) 722-4180

    - Burnsville, St. Louis Park, and St. Paul, Minnesota

        www.emilyprogram.com/locations/minnesota
        (651) 645-5323

- **Healing Minds Specialized Psychotherapy Groups (Philadelphia, Pennsylvania)**

  Women only
  www.healing-minds.com/specializedgroups.html
  (215) 732-1612—Deborah Reeves, MGPGP, CGP, LPC

- **The Howland Way Eating Disorder Recovery Center (Guilford, Connecticut)**

  www.thehowlandway.com/index.html
  (203) 689-5672

- **Inner Door Center (Royal Oak, Michigan)**

  A mindfulness-based treatment approach for men, women, and adolescents
  http://innerdoorcenter.com/index.php/outpatient-clinic
  (248) 336-2868

- **La Ventana (Ventura and Santa Barbara, California)**

  Men, women, and adolescents
  www.laventanaed.com
  www.laventanaed.com/eating-disorder/intensive-outpatient-program/
  (800) 560-8518

- **Linden Oaks (Naperville, Illinois)**

  Women and girls (16 and older)
  www.edward.org/workfiles/eatingdisorders.pdf
  (630) 305-5027

- **McCallum Place (St. Louis, Missouri)**

  Men, women, and adolescents
  www.mccallumplace.com/outpatient-services.html
  (314) 968-1900

- **Mirasol**

  Men, women, and adolescents

www.mirasol.net/treatment-programs/intensive-outpatient-
   program-adult.php
www.mirasol.net/treatment-programs/intensive-outpatient-
   program.php
(888) 520-1700

- **Monte Nido (multiple locations)**

  Men and women
  www.montenido.com
  (310) 457-9958
  Los Angeles, California: http://edcca.com
  Eugene, Oregon: www.rainrock.org/edce-home
  Portland, Oregon: www.rainrock.org/edcp
  Manhattan, New York: www.montenido.com/edtny

- **Rader Programs (Oxnard, California)**

  Men, women, and adolescents
  www.raderprograms.com/treatment/eating-disorder-program.
     html
  www.raderprograms.com/treatment/exercise-therapy.html
  (800) 841-1515

- **Renfrew (multiple locations)**

  Women only
  www.renfrewcenter.com
  (800) RENFREW (736-3739)
  Atlanta, Georgia: http://renfrewcenter.com/locations/non-
     residential/atlanta-ga
  Baltimore, Maryland: http://renfrewcenter.com/locations/non-
     residential/baltimore-md
  Bethesda, Maryland: http://renfrewcenter.com/locations/non-
     residential/bethesda-md
  Boston, Massachussets: http://renfrewcenter.com/locations/all-
     locations/boston-ma
  Brentwood, Tennessee: http://renfrewcenter.com/locations/non-
     residential/brentwood-tn

Charlotte, North Carolina: http://renfrewcenter.com/locations/non-residential/charlotte-nc

Coconut Creek, Florida: http://renfrewcenter.com/locations/non-residential/coconut-creek-fl

Dallas, Texas: http://renfrewcenter.com/locations/non-residential/dallas-tx

Mount Laurel, New Jersey: http://renfrewcenter.com/locations/non-residential/mount-laurel-nj

New York, New York: http://renfrewcenter.com/locations/non-residential/new-york-ny

Old Greenwich, Connecticut: http://renfrewcenter.com/locations/non-residential/old-greenwich-ct

Radnor, Pennsylvania: http://renfrewcenter.com/locations/non-residential/radnor-pa

Ridgewood, New Jersey: http://renfrewcenter.com/locations/non-residential/ridgewood-nj

- **Rogers Memorial Hospital (Madison, West Allis, and Oconomowoc, Wisconsin)**

  Men, women, and adolescents
  http://rogershospital.org/treatment-service/partial-program-adults-and-adolescents
  http://rogershospital.org/treatment-service/partial-program-preteen-young-adults
  (800) 767-4411

- **Shoreline Center for Eating Disorder Treatment (Long Beach and Orange County, California)**

  Men and women
  http://shoreline-eatingdisorders.com
  (562) 434-6007

- **Stone Ridge Healing Arts (Stone Ridge, New York)**

  Men and women
  http://stoneridgehealingarts.com
  (845) 687-7589

- **Tapestry Journeys Day Program (Brevard, North Carolina)**

  Men, women, and adolescents
  www.tapestrync.com/programs/journeys-day-program.html
  (855) 396-2604

- **UNC Center of Excellence for Eating Disorders (Chapel Hill, North Carolina)**

  Men and women
  www.med.unc.edu/psych/eatingdisorders/patient-care-1/partial-
      hospitalization-program
  www.med.unc.edu/psych/eatingdisorders/patient-care-1/
      outpatient-program
  (919) 966-7012

- **Veritas Collaborative (Durham, North Carolina)**

  Adolescent and early adolescent treatment
  http://veritascollaborative.com
  (919) 908-9740

- **The Victory Program at McCallum Place (St. Louis, Missouri)**

  Specifically targeted treatment plans for male and female athletes
  http://thevictoryprogram.com/levels-of-care.html
  (314) 968-1900

- **Webster Wellness Professionals (Webster Groves, Missouri)**

  Men, women, and adolescents
  www.websterwellnessprofessionals.com
  (314) 737-4070

- **Willow Place (multiple locations)**

  Women only
  http://willowplaceforwomen.com

  - Asheville, North Carolina

    http://willowplaceforwomen.com/asheville
    (828) 254-3484

- West Palm Beach, Florida

   http://willowplaceforwomen.com/palm-beach
   (561) 623-0142

- **Woodlands Eating Disorders Center**

   www.woodlandsedc.com
   (281) 465-9229, ext. 100—Dr. Deborah Michelle

FOR FAMILY AND FRIENDS

- **National Association of Anorexia Nervosa and Associated Disorders**

   "How to Help Someone"
   http://www.anad.org/eating-disorders-get-help/how-to-help-a-friend

- **MEDA Parent and Family Support Services**

   http://medainc.org/get-help/parent-and-family-support-services
   (617) 558-1881, ext. 15

- **The Eating Disorder Foundation (Denver, Colorado)**

   Family Connections Support Group, a support group for family and friends
   www.eatingdisorderfoundation.org/Schedule.htm
   (303) 322-3373

- **The Emily Program (multiple locations)**

   Support for family and friends
   www.emilyprogram.com/for-families/family_and_friends
   (651) 645-5323

   Duluth, Minnesota
   St. Paul, Minnesota
   Woodbury, Minnesota
   St. Louis Park, Minnesota
   Seattle, Washington

Spokane, Washington

- **T.H.E. Center Family Support Group (Asheville, North Carolina)**

  http://thecenternc.weebly.com/support-group-schedule.html
  (828) 337-4685

FOR FITNESS PROFESSIONALS

- **Destructively Fit**
  Designed by Jodi Rubin, ACSW, LCSW, CEDS, Destructively Fit is an educational resource that demystifies excessive exercise and eating disorders for personal trainers, group fitness instructors, and others in the fitness industry who wish to better understand and confront unhealthy patterns of physical activity in their clients. Destructively Fit offers in-person and online courses that are endorsed by the American Council on Exercise (ACE) and the National Academy of Sports Medicine (NASM). Trainers and fitness instructors can receive continuing education credits for their completion of Destructively Fit's courses. Rubin is also compiling a referral network of professionals who have undergone Destructively Fit's training. For more information, please visit Destructively Fit's website.
  www.destructivelyfit.com

- Discipio, Laura. "How to Spot and Help Members with Compulsive Exercise or Eating Disorders." *Club Industry.* February 16, 2014. http://clubindustry.com/operations/how-spot-and-help-members-compulsive-exercise-or-eating-disorders.

- Kakaiya, Divya. "Eating Disorders among Athletes." *IDEA Fitness Journal* 5, no. 3 (March 2008). http://www.ideafit.com/fitness-library/eating-disorders-among-athletes.

- Rhew, Jackie, and Robin Boggs Choquette. "Eating Disorders and Athletes: Personality Characteristics and the Parental Support." Alexian Brothers Health System. February 2014. www.cigna.com/assets/

docs/behavioral-health-series/easting-disorder/2014/ed-
and%20athletes-cigna-ed-series-feb-2014.pdf.

- Senger, Megan. "The Tough Stuff: Confronting Clients about Body
  Image–related Health Concerns." *ACE Certified News.*

SUPPORT GROUPS AND NETWORKS

*The following listings offer groups for individuals recovering from pri-
mary or secondary exercise addiction, as well as support networks and
funding resources for those seeking treatment. Please call or visit the
website of the venue or organization you are interested in for further
details regarding times, dates, registration, or application information.*

- **Alexian Brothers Behavioral Health Hospital (Hoffman Es-
  tates, Illinois)**

  www.alexianbrothershealth.org/abbhh/ourservices/eating-
     disorders
  (847) 755-8143

- **ALIVE Center (Bowling Green, Kentucky)**

  www.wku.edu/alive/supportgroup.php
  (270) 535-7653—Sherry Yurchisin

- **ANAD of Baltimore (Baltimore, Maryland)**

  www.ednmaryland.org/upload/ANAD%20flyer[2].pdf
  (410) 440-3074—Sharon R. Peterson, LCSW

- **Aubrey's Song (Owensboro, Kentucky)**

  www.aubreyssong.org
  (270) 233-4445

- **Awakening Center (Chicago, Illinois)**

  http://awakeningcenter.net/calendar.html
  (773) 929-6262 x 15

- **Carolina House (Raleigh, North Carolina)**

  http://carolinahouse.crchealth.com
  (919) 594-6690—Tammy Holcomb, LPC

- **Centennial Counseling Center (Yorkville, Illinois)**

  www.centennialcounseling.com
  (815) 570-9440—Nikki Stepien

- **Eating Disorder Center of Denver (Denver, Colorado)**

  www.edcdenver.com/_literature_64810/Outpatient_Support_
     Group
  (303) 771-0861

- **Eating Disorder Center of San Diego (San Diego, California)**

  http://healingwithinreach.com/adult-group-services
  (858) 353-5378

- **Eating Disorders Resource Center—Body Image & Eating Disorders Support Group (California)**
  The Eating Disorders Resource Center offers multiple free support groups throughout California. Please call or visit their website for the group(s) nearest you.

  www.edrcsv.org/index.php/resources/support-groups.html
  (408) 356-1212

- **Healthy Within (San Diego, California)**
  Healthy Within offers a range of support options for male and female compulsive exercisers and their families. Please call or visit their website to find the right group for you.

  www.healthywithin.com
  (858) 622-0221

- **Insight Psychological Services (Chicago, Illinois)**

  Men and women (17 and older)
  www.insightbhc.com/content/anad-support-group
  (312) 540-9955—Betsy Callan and Sarah Russel

- **Kirsten Haglund Foundation (KHF)**

  Founded by former Miss America pageant winner Kirsten Haglund, KHF helps foster awareness about eating disorders and their accompanying behaviors (like compulsive exercise) and aids in raising funds and scholarships to assist individuals seeking treatment.

  http://kirstenhaglund.com/about-kirsten

- **La Ventana (Thousand Oaks, California)**

  Free support groups offered to men, women, adolescents, friends, and family every day of the week. See website for schedule.

  www.laventanaed.com/about/locations/la-ventana-thousand-oaks
  (805) 777-3873

- **LifeSource (Decatur, Alabama)**

  www.facebook.com/beautifullybroken777
  (256) 341-7403—Shannon Hogan

- **Linden Oaks Outpatient Center (Naperville, Illinois)**

  www.edward.org/BehavioralHealthSupport
  (630) 305-5500

- **MEDA (Newton, Massachusetts)**

  Support groups for men, women, adolescents, and families
  www.medainc.org/get-help/clinical-services
  www.medainc.org/events/calendar
  (617) 558-1881

- **National Association of Anorexia Nervosa and Associated Disorders (ANAD)**

  Founded in 1976, ANAD is a nonprofit organization dedicated to the prevention and treatment of eating disorders and their accompanying symptoms, including overexercise. Its website offers tools for sufferers (including a confidential help hotline) as well as for individuals concerned about loved ones struggling with body image disorders or exercise addiction.

  www.anad.org

www.anad.org/eating-disorders-get-help/eating-disorders-
   support-groups
630-577-1330

- **National Eating Disorders Association (NEDA)**

   *NEDA helps individuals suffering from secondary exercise addic-
   tion and eating disorders find treatment and other resources to aid
   them in their recovery process. Their website offers free screening
   tools in addition to a nationwide list of inpatient, outpatient, and
   group therapy programs for those grappling with body image,
   weight, and abuses of exercise or food. Their helpline, listed below, is
   open Monday through Thursday from 9:00 am to 9:00 pm and Fri-
   days from 9:00 am until 5:00 pm. Through their support network of
   "navigators," NEDA also connects sufferers looking to recover with
   individuals who have themselves overcome eating disorders or overexercise.*

   www.nationaleatingdisorders.org/find-treatment/support-groups-
      research-studies
   (800) 931-2237

- **Overcoming Eating Disorders ANAD Support Group (San
   Francisco, California)**

   www.overcomingeatingdisorderstherapy.com/free_ANAD_
      Support_Group.html
   (415) 640-9862

- **Positive Pathways (Denver, Colorado)**

   www.positivepathways.com/new/Groups_%26_Workshops.html
   (303) 494-1975

- **Project HEAL**

   *Founded by two women who met while undergoing treatment for
   their own eating disorders, Project HEAL is a nonprofit organization
   devoted to raising funds to assist individuals seeking treatment for
   self-destructive relationships with exercise and/or food across the
   United States and Canada. Project HEAL offers a number of re-*

sources for sufferers and their loved ones, including educational tools and treatment options.

www.theprojectheal.org

- **Prosperity Wellness Center (Herndon, Virginia)**

    www.prosperityedwell.com
    www.prosperityedwell.com/iop-group-calendar
    (703) 466-5150

- **Quad Cities Eating Disorders Support Group (Davenport, Iowa)**

    www.unitypoint.org/quadcities/services-get-help.aspx
    (563) 742-5800—Trinity Enrichment Center
    (309) 786-3006—Betsy Zmuda-Swanson, LCSW (facilitator)

- **Sheena's Place (Toronto, Canada)**
    Sheena's Place is a support center for those with body image issues located in Toronto, Canada. Founded by Lynn Carpenter, the mother of Sheena Carpenter, a young woman who died as a consequence of her anorexia, Sheena's Place offers group support, education, and awareness programs about eating disorders and compulsive exercise in the interest of better informing the public and assisting women, men, and their loved ones in the recovery process.

    www.sheenasplace.org
    416-927-8900

- **Stable Wellness (Lexington, Kentucky)**

    Positive body image groups and camp programs for girls
    www.StableWellness.com
    (859) 948-8644

- **Stone Ridge Healing Arts (Stone Ridge, New York)**

    Men and women
    http://stoneridgehealingarts.com
    (845) 687-7589

- **T.H.E. Center Adult Support Group (Asheville, North Carolina)**

  Men, women, and adolescents
  http://thecenternc.weebly.com/support-group-schedule.html
  (828) 337-4685

- **The Eating Disorder Foundation (Denver, Colorado)**

  www.eatingdisorderfoundation.org/Schedule.htm
  (303) 322-3373

- **The Emily Program (St. Paul, Minnesota)**

  Recovery Night
  www.emilyprogram.com/for-you/recovery_night
  (651) 645-5323

- **The F.R.E.E.D. Foundation**
  The Gail R. Schoenbach F.R.E.E.D. Foundation is a nonprofit organization devoted to raising money to assist individuals seeking treatment for eating disorders and their accompanying behaviors. The F.R.E.E.D. Foundation also backs education and awareness endeavors by scheduling speaking opportunities and furthering activist efforts related to body image issues.

  www.freedfoundation.org

- **The Joy Project Support Group (Minneapolis, Minnesota)**

  http://joyproject.org/628/support-group
  (651) 334-0368

- **The Manna Fund**
  The Manna Fund is a nonprofit organization geared toward financially assisting individuals seeking treatment for body image issues, eating disorders, and compulsive exercise.

  www.mannafund.org

- **The National Association for Males with Eating Disorders (N.A.M.E.D.)**

http://namedinc.org

- **UNC Center of Excellence for Eating Disorders (Chapel Hill, North Carolina)**

    Outpatient group therapy for adults and adolescents
    www.med.unc.edu/psych/eatingdisorders/patient-care-1/group-
        therapies
    (919) 966-7012

- **Valley Village and Encino ANAD Support Group (Valley Village, California)**

    http://therapyhelps.us/groups
    (818) 388-2355

- **Woodlands Eating Disorders Center (The Woodlands, Texas)**

    www.woodlandsedc.com
    (281) 465-9229

HEALTHIER EXERCISE PROGRAMS AND ALTERNATIVES

- **Awakening Center**

    *For additional group support and alternative therapies, please call
        or visit the Awakening Center's website.*
    www.awakeningcenter.net
    (773) 929-6262—Mari Richko (Yoga Talk Group)

- **MovNat**

    www.movnat.com

- **Nia Technique**

    www.nianow.com/find/classes

- **Positive Pathways (Denver, Colorado)**

    Intuitive exercise program
    www.positivepathways.com/new/ED_%26_Athletes.html

(720) 301-1752

- **The Howland Way (Guilford, Connecticut)**

  http://www.thehowlandway.com/index.html

APPENDIX B

Common Exercise Addiction Measures

Several measurement tools exist that attempt to quantify various aspects of exercise addiction. Each tool has its own advantages and disadvantages in measuring facets of addiction that are pertinent to either general or specific populations[1] (e.g., eating-disordered individuals, bodybuilders). We have included the following three commonly used exercise addiction measures that have also demonstrated superior psychometrics and present an approach to quantifying exercise addiction that may be broadly applicable to multiple fields of research:[2]

- Exercise Addiction Inventory (EAI)
- Exercise Dependence Scale (EDS)
- Compulsive Exercise Test (CET)

EXERCISE ADDICTION INVENTORY

Designed by behavioral addiction researchers Annabel Terry, Attila Szabó, and Mark D. Griffiths, the EAI[3] is a quick and simple screening tool measure that is based on theoretical constructs of behavioral addiction.[4] The EAI includes one item for each of the following six components of behavioral addiction:

- Salience ("Exercise is the most important thing in my life.")
- Mood modification ("I use exercise as a way of changing my mood.")
- Tolerance ("Over time I have increased the amount of exercise I do in a day.")
- Withdrawal ("If I have to miss an exercise session, I feel moody and irritable.")
- Conflict ("Conflicts have arisen between me and my family and/or my partner about the amount of exercise I do.")
- Relapse ("If I cut down on the amount of exercise I do and then start again, I always end up exercising as often as I did before.")

Responses to the items are on a five-point Likert scale ranging from 1 (strongly disagree) to 5 (strongly agree). Item scores are summed and higher total scores reflect problematic exercise. The EAI can also be used categorically. Total scores of 0–12 are indicative of an "asymptomatic individual." Scores of 13–23 are indicative of a "symptomatic individual." Scores above 24 are indicative of an "at-risk of exercise addiction individual." A cutoff score of 24 reflects the top 15 percent of responses.[5]

Exercise Addiction Inventory

Instructions: Listed below are a series of statements regarding exercise. Please read each statement carefully and indicate the number that best indicates how true each statement is of you. Please answer all the questions as honestly as you can.

1 Strongly Disagree	2	3 Neither Agree nor Disagree	4	5 Strongly Agree

1. Exercise is the most important thing in my life. _____
2. I use exercise as a way of changing my mood (e.g., to get a buzz, to escape). _____
3. Over time I have increased the amount of exercise I do in a day. _____
4. If I have to miss an exercise session, I feel moody and irritable. _____

5. Conflicts have arisen between me and my family and/or me and my partner about the amount of exercise I do. _____
6. If I cut down on the amount of exercise I do and then start again, I always end up exercising as often as I did before. _____

EXERCISE DEPENDENCE SCALE

Created by exercise addiction researchers Heather Hausenblas and Danielle Symons Downs, the EDS[6] is a twenty-one-item measure of exercise dependence symptoms that was developed to reflect the criteria for substance dependence listed in the fourth edition of the American Psychiatric Association's *Diagnostic and Statistical Manual of Mental Disorders (DSM-IV)*. The EDS includes seven subscales consisting of three items each that assess:

- Tolerance (e.g., "I continually increase my exercise frequency to achieve the desired effects/benefits.")
- Withdrawal effects (e.g., "I exercise to avoid feeling tense.")
- Continuance (e.g., "I exercise despite persistent physical problems.")
- Lack of control (e.g., "I am unable to reduce how intense I exercise.")
- Reductions in other activities (e.g., "I think about exercise when I should be concentrating on school/work.")
- Time (e.g., "I spend a lot of time exercising.")
- Intention (e.g., "I exercise longer than I expect.")

Responses to the items are on a six-point Likert scale ranging from 1 (never) to 6 (always). A lower score reveals fewer exercise dependence symptoms. Responses can be summed for a total continuous score of exercise dependence symptoms. Additionally, the scale can be used categorically. Individuals endorsing scores of five to six on items for at least three subscales are categorized as "at-risk for exercise dependence"; scores of three to four on at least three subscales are categorized as "nondependent symptomatic"; and scores of one to two are categorized as "nondependent asymptomatic." The psychometric properties of this scale are accurate.[7] This scale has not yet been updated to reflect the recent addition of cravings in the substance use disorder criteria in the most recent edition of the *DSM (DSM-V)*.

Exercise Dependence Scale

Instructions: Using the scale provided below, please complete the following questions as honestly as possible. The questions refer to current exercise beliefs and behaviors that have occurred in the *past three months*. Please write your answer in the blank space provided after each statement.

1 Never	2	3	4	5	6 Always

1. I exercise to avoid feeling irritable. _____
2. I exercise despite recurring physical problems. _____
3. I continually increase my exercise intensity to achieve the desired effects/benefits. _____
4. I am unable to reduce how long I exercise. _____
5. I would rather exercise than spend time with family/friends. _____
6. I spend a lot of time exercising. _____
7. I exercise longer than I intend. _____
8. I exercise to avoid feeling anxious. _____
9. I exercise when injured. _____
10. I continually increase my exercise frequency to achieve the desired effects/benefits. _____
11. I am unable to reduce how often I exercise. _____
12. I think about exercise when I should be concentrating on school/work. _____
13. I spend most of my free time exercising. _____
14. I exercise longer than I expect. _____
15. I exercise to avoid feeling tense. _____
16. I exercise despite persistent physical problems. _____
17. I continually increase my exercise duration to achieve the desired effects/benefits. _____
18. I am unable to reduce how intensely I exercise. _____
19. I choose to exercise so that I can avoid spending time with family/friends. _____

20. A great deal of my time is spent exercising. _____
21. I exercise longer than I plan. _____

Scoring:

Component	Item Numbers
Withdrawal effects	1, 8, 15
Continuance	2, 9, 16
Tolerance	3, 10, 17
Lack of control	4, 11, 18
Reduction in other activities	5, 12, 19
Time	6, 13, 20
Intention effects	7, 14, 21

COMPULSIVE EXERCISE TEST

The CET,[8] designed by psychologists Lorin Taranis, Stephen Touyz, and Caroline Meyer, is a twenty-four-item self-report measure that assesses compulsive features of exercise that are implicated in the maintenance of excessive exercise in eating disorders. The CET includes the following five subscales:

- Avoidance and rule-driven behavior (e.g., "I usually continue to exercise despite injury.")
- Weight control exercise (e.g., "I exercise to burn calories and lose weight.")
- Mood improvement (e.g., "I feel less anxious after I exercise.")
- Lack of exercise enjoyment (e.g., "I find exercise a chore.")
- Exercise rigidity (e.g., "My weekly pattern of exercise is repetitive.")

The Compulsive Exercise Test uses a six-point Likert scale anchored by 0 (never true) and 5 (always true) with higher scores indicative of greater pathology. An item on the "weight control exercise" subscale is reverse scored (e.g., "I do not exercise to be slim")—as is an item on the "lack of exercise enjoyment" subscale (e.g., "I enjoy exercising"). All items may then be summed to provide a total score. Items included in each subscale may also be summed. The CET has demonstrated good psychometric properties.[9]

CET Scoring Criteria:

- Items 8 and 12 are reverse scored.
- Subscale scores are obtained by summing the scores for all items in the subscale and dividing by the number of items (mean score).
- CET total score is calculated by summing the mean scores for all subscales.

Subscale Items:

- Avoidance and rule-driven behavior: 9, 10, 11, 15, 16, 20, 22, 23
- Weight control exercise: 2, 6, 8, 13, 18
- Mood improvement: 1, 4, 14, 17, 24
- Lack of exercise enjoyment: 5, 12, 21
- Exercise rigidity: 3, 7, 19

Compulsive Exercise Test

Instructions: Listed below are a series of statements regarding exercise. Please read each statement carefully and indicate the number that best indicates how true each statement is of you. Please answer all the questions as honestly as you can.

0	1	2	3	4	5
Never True	Rarely True	Sometimes True	Often True	Usually True	Always True

1. I feel happier and/or more positive after I exercise. _____
2. I exercise to improve my appearance. _____
3. I like my days to be organized and structured, of which exercise is just one part. _____

4. I feel less anxious after I exercise. _____
5. I find exercise a chore. _____
6. If I feel I have eaten too much, I will do more exercise. _____
7. My weekly pattern of exercise is repetitive. _____
8. I do not exercise to be slim. _____
9. If I cannot exercise I feel low or depressed. _____
10. I feel extremely guilty if I miss an exercise session. _____
11. I usually continue to exercise despite injury or illness, unless I am very ill or too injured. _____
12. I enjoy exercising. _____
13. I exercise to burn calories and to lose weight. _____
14. I feel less stressed and/or tense after I exercise. _____
15. If I miss an exercise session, I will try and make up for it when I next exercise. _____
16. If I cannot exercise I feel agitated and/or irritable. _____
17. Exercise improves my mood. _____
18. If I cannot exercise, I worry that I will gain weight. _____
19. I follow a set routine for my exercise sessions (e.g., walk or run the same route, perform particular exercises, exercise for the same amount of time, and so on). _____
20. If I cannot exercise I feel angry and/or frustrated. _____
21. I do not enjoy exercising. _____
22. I feel like I've let myself down if I miss an exercise session. _____
23. If I cannot exercise I feel anxious. _____
24. I feel less depressed or low after I exercise. _____

NOTES

I. WHAT IT IS

1. Steve Sussman, Nadra Lisha, and Mark Griffiths, "Prevalence of the Addictions: A Problem of the Majority or the Minority?" *Evaluation & the Health Professions* 34, no. 1 (2011): 3–56, DOI:10.1177/0163278710380124.

2. Krisztina Berczik, Attila Szabó, Mark D. Griffiths, Tamás Kurimay, Bernadette Kun, Róbert Urbán, and Zsolt Demetrovics, "Exercise Addiction: Symptoms, Diagnosis, Epidemiology, and Etiology," *Substance Use & Misuse* 47, no. 4 (2012): 403–17, DOI:10.3109/10826084.2011.639120.

3. Kata Mónok, Krisztina Berczik, Róbert Urbán, Attila Szabó, Mark D. Griffiths, Judit Farkas, Anna Magi, Andrea Eisinger, Tamás Kurimay, Gyöngyi Kökönyei, Bernadette Kun, Borbála Paski, and Zsolt Demetrovics, "Psychometric Properties and Concurrent Validity of Two Exercise Addiction Measures: A Population Wide Study," *Psychology of Sport and Exercise* 13, no. 6 (2012): 739–46, DOI:10.1016/j.psychsport.2012.06.003.

4. Heather A. Slay, Jumi Hayaki, Melissa A. Napolitano, and Kelly D. Brownell, "Motivations for Running and Eating Attitudes in Obligatory versus Nonobligatory Runners," *International Journal of Eating Disorders* 23, no. 3 (1998): 267–75, DOI:10.1002/(SICI)1098-108X(199804)23:3&#60267::AID-EAT4&#623.0.CO;2-H.

5. Michelle J. Blaydon and Koenraad J. Lindner, "Eating Disorders and Exercise Dependence in Triathletes," *Eating Disorders* 10, no. 1 (2002): 49–60, DOI:10.1080/106402602753573559.

6. Sebastiano Costa, Heather A. Hausenblas, Patrizia Oliva, Francesca Cuzzocrea, and Rosalba Larcan, "The Role of Age, Gender, Mood States and

Exercise Frequency on Exercise Dependence," *Journal of Behavioral Addictions* 2, no. 4 (2013): 216–23, DOI:10.1556/JBA.2.2013.014.

7. Kata Mónok, Krisztina Berczik, Róbert Urbán, Attila Szabó, Mark D. Griffiths, Judit Farkas, Anna Magi, Andrea Eisinger, Tamás Kurimay, Gyöngyi Kökönyei, Bernadette Kun, Borbála Paksi, and Zsolt Demetrovics, "Psychometric Properties and Concurrent Validity of Two Exercise Addiction Measures: A Population Wide Study," *Psychology of Sport and Exercise* 13, no. 6 (2012): 739–46, DOI:10.1016/j.psychsport.2012.06.003.

8. Steve Sussman, Nadra Lisha, and Mark Griffiths, "Prevalence of the Addictions: A Problem of the Majority or the Minority?" *Evaluation & the Health Professions* 34, no. 1 (2011): 3–56, DOI:10.1177/0163278710380124.

9. Sandy Baum, Jennifer Ma, and Kathleen Payea, "Health Benefits: Exercise," *Education Pays 2013: The Benefits of Higher Education for Individuals and Society* (New York: The College Board, 2013), 28.

10. Lisa M. Powell, Sandy Slater, and Frank J. Chaloupka, "The Relationship between Community Physical Activity Settings and Race, Ethnicity and Socioeconomic Status," *Evidence-Based Prevention Medicine* 1, no. 2 (2004): 135–44.

11. Heather A. Hausenblas and Danielle Symons Downs, "Exercise Dependence: A Systematic Review," *Psychology of Sport and Exercise* 3, no. 2 (2002): 89–123, DOI:10.1016/S1469-0292(00)00015-7.

12. Heather A. Hausenblas and Danielle Symons Downs, "Exercise Dependence: A Systematic Review," *Psychology of Sport and Exercise* 3, no. 2 (2002): 89–123, DOI:10.1016/S1469-0292(00)00015-7.

13. Aviel Goodman, "Neurobiology of Addiction: An Integrative Review," *Biochemical Pharmacology* 75, no. 1 (2008): 266–322, DOI:10.1016/j.bcp.2007.07.030.

14. Alayne Yates, *Compulsive Exercise and the Eating Disorders* (New York: Brunner/Mazel, 1991).

15. Diane A. Klein, Andrew S. Bennett, Janet Schebendach, Richard W. Foltin, Michael J. Devlin, and B. Timothy Walsh, "Exercise 'Addiction' in Anorexia Nervosa: Model Development and Pilot Data," *CNS Spectrums* 9, no. 7 (2004): 531–37.

16. Brian Cook, Trisha M. Karr, Christie Zunker, James E. Mitchell, Ron Thompson, Roberta Sherman, Ross D. Crosby, Li Cao, Ann Erickson, and Stephen A. Wonderlich, "Primary and Secondary Exercise Dependence in a Community-based Sample of Road Race Runners," *Journal of Sport & Exercise Psychology* 35, no. 5 (2013): 464–69.

17. American Psychiatric Association, *Diagnostic and Statistical Manual of Mental Disorders* (Washington, DC: American Psychiatric Association, 2013).

2. WHAT IT LOOKS LIKE

1. Arnaud Merglen, Aline Flatz, Richard E. Bélanger, Pierre-André Michaud, and Joan-Carles Suris, "Weekly Sport Practice and Adolescent Well-being," *Archives of Disease in Childhood* 99, no. 3 (2013): 208–10, DOI:10.1136/archdischild-2013-303729.

2. Cheryl J. Hansen, Larry C. Stevens, and Richard J. Coast, "Exercise Duration and Mood State: How Much Is Enough to Feel Better?" *Health Psychology* 20, no. 4 (2001): 267–75, DOI:10.1037/0278-6133.20.4.267.

3. Heather A. Hausenblas and Danielle Symons Downs, "Exercise Dependence: A Systematic Review," *Psychology of Sport and Exercise* 3, no. 2 (2002): 89–123, DOI:10.1016/S1469-0292(00)00015-7.

4. Heather A. Hausenblas and Danielle Symons Downs, "Exercise Dependence: A Systematic Review," *Psychology of Sport and Exercise* 3, no. 2 (2002): 89–123, DOI:10.1016/S1469-0292(00)00015-7.

5. Attila Szabó, "The Impact of Exercise Deprivation on Well-being of Habitual Exercisers," *Australian Journal of Science and Medicine in Sport* 27, no. 3 (1995): 68–75.

6. Marita P. McCabe and Lina A. Ricciardelli, "Body Image Dissatisfaction among Males across the Lifespan: A Review of Past Literature," *Journal of Psychosomatic Research* 56, no. 6 (2004): 675–85, DOI:10.1016/S0022-3999(03)00129-6.

7. David de Coverley Veale, "Exercise Dependence," *British Journal of Addiction* 82, no. 7 (1987): 735–40, DOI:10.1111/j.1360-0443.1987.tb01539. x.

8. Alayne Yates, *Compulsive Exercise and the Eating Disorders* (New York: Brunner/Mazel, 1991), 58.

9. Justin McNamara and Marita P. McCabe, "Striving for Success or Addiction? Exercise Dependence among Elite Australian Athletes," *Journal of Sports Sciences* 30, no. 8 (2012): 755–66, DOI:10.1080/02640414.2012.667879.

10. Lorin Taranis and Caroline Meyer, "Associations between Specific Components of Compulsive Exercise and Eating-disordered Cognitions and Behaviors among Young Women," *The International Journal of Eating Disorders* 44, no. 5 (2011): 452–58, DOI:10.1002/eat.20838.

11. Alayne Yates, *Compulsive Exercise and the Eating Disorders* (New York: Brunner/Mazel, 1991).

12. Alayne Yates, *Compulsive Exercise and the Eating Disorders* (New York: Brunner/Mazel, 1991).

13. Christopher Fairburn, Zafra Cooper, and Roz Shafran, "Cognitive Behaviour Therapy for Eating Disorders: A 'Transdiagnostic' Theory and Treat-

ment," *Behaviour Research and Therapy* 41, no. 5 (2003): 509–28, DOI:10.1016/S0005-7967(02)00088-8.

14. Lorin Taranis and Caroline Meyer, "Associations between Specific Components of Compulsive Exercise and Eating-disordered Cognitions and Behaviors among Young Women," *The International Journal of Eating Disorders* 44, no. 5 (2011): 452–58, DOI:10.1002/eat.20838.

15. Jonathan M. Mond, Phillipa J. Hay, Bryan Rodgers, and Cathy Owen, "An Update on the Definition of 'Excessive Exercise' in Eating Disorders Research," *International Journal of Eating Disorders* 39, no. 2 (2006): 147–53, DOI:10.1002/eat.20214.

16. Jonathan M. Mond and Rachel M. Calogero, "Excessive Exercise in Eating Disorder Patients and Healthy Women," *Australian and New Zealand Journal of Psychiatry* 43, no. 3 (2009): 227–34, DOI:10.1080/00048670802653323.

17. Jonathan M. Mond, Tricia C. Myers, Ross Crosby, Phillipa Hay, and James Mitchell, "Excessive Exercise and Eating-disordered Behaviour in Young Adult Women: Further Evidence from a Primary Care Sample," *European Eating Disorders Review* 16, no. 3 (2008): 215–21, DOI:10.1002/erv.855.

18. Clive G. Long, Jenny Smith, Marie Midgley, and Tony Cassidy, "Over-exercising in Anorexic and Normal Samples: Behaviour and Attitudes," *Journal of Mental Health* 2, no. 4 (1993): 321–27, DOI:10.3109/09638239309016967.

19. Eva Peñas-Lledó, Francisco J. Vaz Leal, and Glen Waller, "Excessive Exercise in Anorexia Nervosa and Bulimia Nervosa: Relation to Eating Characteristics and General Psychopathology," *International Journal of Eating Disorders* 31, no. 4 (2002): 370–75, DOI:10.1002/eat.10042.

20. Lori A. Goldfarb, Elisabeth M. Dykens, and Meg Gerrard, "The Goldfarb Fear of Fat Scale," *Journal of Personality Assessment* 49, no. 3 (1985): 329–32, DOI:10.1207/s15327752jpa4903_21.

21. Brian Cook, Heather Hausenblas, Daniel Tuccitto, and Peter R. Giacobbi, "Eating Disorders and Exercise: A Structural Equation Modeling Analysis of a Conceptual Model," *European Eating Disorders Review* 19, no. 3 (2011): 216–25, DOI:10.1002/erv.1111.

3. WHO COINED IT?

1. Kenneth John Freeman, *Schools of Hellas: An Essay on the Practice and Theory of Ancient Greek Education from 600 to 300 B.C.* (London: St. Martin's Press, 1907), 119.

2. Kenneth John Freeman, *Schools of Hellas: An Essay on the Practice and Theory of Ancient Greek Education from 600 to 300 B.C.* (London: St. Martin's Press, 1907), 120.

3. Xenophon, *Hellenica*, c. 370 BC, quoted in Stephen G. Miller, *Arete: Greek Sports from Ancient Sources* (Berkeley: University of California Press, 1991), 184.

4. Paul Christesen and Donald G. Kyle, *A Companion to Sport and Spectacle in Greek and Roman Antiquity* (Malden, MA: Wiley-Blackwell, 2014), 609.

5. Xenophon, *Memorabilia*, c. 371 BC, quoted in E. Norman Gardiner, *Athletics in the Ancient World* (London: Oxford University Press, 1930), 71.

6. Nigel B. Crowther, *Sport in Ancient Times* (Westport, CT: Praeger Publications, 2007), 76.

7. Kenneth John Freeman, *Schools of Hellas: An Essay on the Practice and Theory of Ancient Greek Education from 600 to 300 B.C.* (London: St. Martin's Press, 1907), 122.

8. Paul Christesen and Donald G. Kyle, *A Companion to Sport and Spectacle in Greek and Roman Antiquity* (Malden, MA: Wiley-Blackwell, 2014), 608.

9. *Exhortation to Study the Arts* 11, trans. Konig 2005: 296, in Paul Christesen and Donald G. Kyle, *A Companion to Sport and Spectacle in Greek and Roman Antiquity* (Malden, MA: Wiley-Blackwell, 2014), 608.

10. Daryl Siedentop, *Introduction to Physical Education, Fitness, and Sport*, 7th ed. (New York: McGraw-Hill Higher Education, 2009), chap. 2; http://highered.mcgraw-hill.com/sites/dl/free/0073376515/669664/Siedentop7e_ch02.pdf (accessed February 24, 2014).

11. John McClelland, *Body and Mind: Sport in Europe from the Roman Empire to the Renaissance* (New York: Routledge, 2007), 22.

12. Daniel McLean and Amy Hurd, *Kraus' Recreation and Leisure in Modern Society* (Burlington, MA: Jones & Bartlett Learning, 2012), 35–85.

13. David Kirk, Doune Macdonald, and Mary O'Sullivan, *Handbook of Physical Education* (London: Sage, 2006), 128.

14. William H. Freeman, *Physical Education, Exercise and Sport Science in a Changing Society*, 7th ed. (Burlington, MA: Jones & Bartlett Learning, 2012), chap. 4.

15. Thierry Terret and J. A. Mangan, *Sport, Militarism and the Great War* (New York: Routledge, 2012), 16.

16. David Kirk, Doune Macdonald, and Mary O'Sullivan, *Handbook of Physical Education* (London: Sage, 2006), 128.

17. Murray G. Phillips and Alexander Paul Roper, "History of Physical Education," in *Handbook of Physical Education*, ed. David Kirk, Doune Macdon-

ald, and Mary O'Sullivan (Burlington, MA: Jones & Bartlett Learning, 2015), 123–41.

18. Robert A. Mechikoff and Stephen Estes, *A History and Philosophy of Sport and Physical Education*, 3rd ed. (Boston: McGraw Hill, 2002), 119.

19. William H. Freeman, *Physical Education, Exercise and Sport Science in a Changing Society*, 7th ed. (Burlington, MA: Jones & Bartlett Learning, 2012), 101–2.

20. William H. Freeman, *Physical Education, Exercise and Sport Science in a Changing Society*, 7th ed. (Burlington, MA: Jones & Bartlett Learning, 2012), 123–24.

21. William H. Freeman, *Physical Education, Exercise and Sport Science in a Changing Society*, 7th ed. (Burlington, MA: Jones & Bartlett Learning, 2012), 100–104.

22. William H. Freeman, *Physical Education, Exercise and Sport Science in a Changing Society*, 7th ed. (Burlington, MA: Jones & Bartlett Learning, 2012), 107.

23. Robert A. Mechikoff and Stephen Estes, *A History and Philosophy of Sport and Physical Education*, 3rd ed. (Boston: McGraw Hill, 2002), 164.

24. William H. Freeman, *Physical Education, Exercise and Sport Science in a Changing Society*, 7th ed. (Burlington, MA: Jones & Bartlett Learning, 2012), 108.

25. Clifford Putney, *Muscular Christianity: Manhood and Sports in Protestant America, 1880–1920* (Cambridge, MA: Harvard University Press, 2001).

26. Anonymous, "Athletics in Schools," *The Popular Science Monthly* 16 (March 1880): 677–84.

27. Julie Hepworth, *The Social Construction of Anorexia Nervosa* (London: Sage, 1999), 26.

28. William Gull, "Anorexia Nervosa (Apepsia Hysteria)," *Transactions of the Clinical Society of London* 7 (1874): 22–28.

29. Max Wallet, "Deux cas d'anorexie hystérique," in *Nouvelle Iconographie de la Salpêtrière*, ed. J.-M. Charcot (Paris, 1892), 278.

30. Pierre Janet, *The Major Symptoms of Hysteria: Fifteen Lectures Given in the Medical School of Harvard University* (London: Macmillan, 1920).

31. Clifford Putney, *Muscular Christianity: Manhood and Sports in Protestant America, 1880–1920* (Cambridge, MA: Harvard University Press, 2001).

32. Peter Hayward, *Intermediate GNVQ Leisure and Tourism Student Book without Options* (Oxford: Heinemann Educational Publishers, 2000), 5.

33. Shelly McKenzie, *Getting Physical: The Rise of Fitness Culture in America* (Lawrence: University Press of Kansas, 2013).

34. Jennifer Smith Maguire, "Body Lessons: Fitness Publishing and the Cultural Production of the Fitness Consumer," *International Review for the*

Sociology of Sport 37, nos. 3–4 (2002): 449–64, DOI:10.1177/
1012690202037004896.

35. Shelly McKenzie, *Getting Physical: The Rise of Fitness Culture in America* (Lawrence: University Press of Kansas, 2013).

36. Sharon Zukin and Jennifer Smith Maguire, "Consumers and Consumption," *Annual Review of Sociology* 30 (2004): 173–97, DOI:10.1146/annurev.soc.30.012703.110553.

37. Pierre Bourdieu, *Distinction: A Social Critique of the Judgment of Taste* (Cambridge, MA: Harvard University Press, 1984).

38. Jennifer Smith Maguire, "Body Lessons: Fitness Publishing and the Cultural Production of the Fitness Consumer," *International Review for the Sociology of Sport* 37, nos. 3–4 (2002): 449–64, DOI:10.1177/
1012690202037004896.

39. Frederick Baekeland, "Exercise Deprivation: Sleep and Psychological Reactions," *Archives of General Psychiatry* 22, no. 4 (1970): 365–69, DOI:10.1001/archpsyc.1970.01740280077014.

40. Howard Padwa and Jacob Cunningham, *Addiction: A Reference Encyclopedia* (Santa Barbara, CA: Greenwood Publishing Group, 2010), 224.

41. National Counsel on Alcoholism, "Criteria for the Diagnosis of Alcoholism," *American Journal of Psychiatry* 129, no. 2 (1972): 127–35.

42. Grischa Metlay, "Federalizing Medical Campaigns against Alcoholism and Drug Abuse," *Milbank Quarterly* 91, no. 1 (2013): 123–62, DOI:10.1111/
milq.12004.

43. William P. Morgan, "Negative Addiction in Runners," *Physician and Sportsmedicine* 7, no. 7 (1979): 57–70.

44. David De Coverley Veale, "Exercise Dependence," *British Journal of Addiction* 82, no. 7 (1987): 735–40, DOI:10.1111/j.1360-0443.1987.tb01539.x.

45. William Glasser, *Positive Addictions* (New York: Harper Colophon, 1976).

46. William P. Morgan, "Negative Addiction in Runners," *Physician and Sportsmedicine* 7, no. 7 (1979): 57–70.

47. Anna Aarenstein, "Home Fitness Reaches Mind-boggling Sales Explosion," *Gainesville Sun*, June 24, 1984.

48. Gale Group, "Physical Fitness Facilities SIC 7991 Industry Reports," *Highbeam Business Report*, http://business.highbeam.com/industry-reports/
personal/physical-fitness-facilities (accessed February 24, 2014).

49. International Health, Racquet, and Sportsclub Association, "Consumer Research," www.ihrsa.org/consumer-research (accessed February 24, 2014).

50. The CDC's current physical activity guidelines for adults recommend a minimum of 150 weekly minutes of moderately strenuous aerobic activity (think: walking fast enough to make a train on time) and two bouts of muscle-

strengthening exercises targeting all major muscle groups per week. (For the fitter among us, an hour and fifteen minutes spent jogging or pumping our heart rates to the max on a cardio machine also fulfills the aerobic requirement.) Kids, by contrast, should remain active for one hour each day.

51. Centers for Disease Control and Prevention, "How Much Physical Activity Do You Need?" www.cdc.gov/physicalactivity/everyone/guidelines/index.html (accessed April 23, 2014).

52. International Health, Racquet, and Sportsclub Association, *The Global Report*, 2013, 32.

53. International Health, Racquet, and Sportsclub Association, *The Global Report*, 2013, 33.

54. International Health, Racquet, and Sportsclub Association, *The Global Report*, 2013, 32.

55. International Health, Racquet, and Sportsclub Association, *The Global Report*, 2013, 32.

56. International Health, Racquet, and Sportsclub Association, *The Global Report*, 2013, 32.

57. International Health, Racquet, and Sportsclub Association, *The Global Report*, 2013, 32.

58. International Health, Racquet, and Sportsclub Association, "Global Health Club Industry Proves Resilient," *The Global Report*, 2013, 9.

59. International Health, Racquet, and Sportsclub Association, *The Global Report*, 2013, 33.

60. International Health, Racquet, and Sportsclub Association, *The Global Report*, 2013, 33.

61. Anonymous, "The Cult of the Gym: The New Puritans," *The Economist*, December 19, 2002, www.economist.com/node/1487649 (accessed February 24, 2014).

4. HOW IT BEGINS

1. George E. Barnes, Robert P. Murray, David Patton, Peter M. Bentler, and Robert E. Anderson, *The Addiction-prone Personality* (New York: Kluwer Academic/Plenum Publishers, 2000).

2. Harvard Health Publications, "The Addicted Brain," *Harvard Mental Health Letter*, July 2004, www.health.harvard.edu/newsweek/The_addicted_brain.htm (accessed February 22, 2014).

3. Christine Sarramon, Hélène Verdoux, Laurent Schmitt, and Marc-Louis Bourgeois, "Addiction and Personality Traits: Sensation Seeking, Anhedonia, Impulsivity," *L'Encéphale* 25, no. 6 (1999): 569–75.

4. Rajita Sinha, "Chronic Stress, Drug Use, and Vulnerability to Addiction," *Annals of the New York Academy of Sciences* 1141 (2008): 105–30, DOI:10.1196/annals.1441.030.

5. Elaine Setiawan, Robert O. Pihl, Alain Dagher, Hera Schlagintweit, Kevin F. Casey, Chawki Benkelfat, and Marco Leyton, "Differential Striatal Dopamine Responses Following Oral Alcohol in Individuals at Varying Risk for Dependence," *Alcoholism: Clinical and Experimental Research* 38, no. 1 (2014): 126–34, DOI:10.1111/acer.12218.

6. David E. Smith, "Editor's Note: The Process Addictions and the New ASAM Definition of Addiction," *Journal of Psychoactive Drugs* 44, no. 1 (2012): 1–4, DOI:10.1080/02791072.2012.662105.

7. Aviel Goodman, "Neurobiology of Addiction: An Integrative Review," *Biochemical Pharmacology* 75, no. 1 (2008): 266–322, DOI:10.1016/j.bcp.2007.07.030.

8. Charles H. Hillman, Kirk I. Erickson, and Arthur F. Kramer, "Be Smart, Exercise Your Heart: Exercise Effects on Brain and Cognition," *Nature Reviews Neuroscience* 9, no. 1 (2008): 58–65, DOI:10.1038/nrn2298.

9. Kirk I. Erickson, Michelle W. Vossb, Ruchika Shaurya Prakash, Chandramallika Basak, Attila Szabó, Laura Chaddock, Jennifer S. Kim, Susie Heo, Heloisa Alves, Siobhan M. White, Thomas R. Wojcicki, Emily Mailey, Victoria J. Vieira, Stephen A. Martin, Brandt D. Pence, Jeffrey A. Woods, Edward McAuley, and Arthur F. Kramer, "Exercise Training Increases Size of Hippocampus and Improves Memory," *Proceedings of the National Academy of Sciences* 108, no. 7 (2011): 3017–22, DOI:10.1073/pnas.1015950108.

10. Janet Buckworth, Rod K. Dishman, Patrick J. O'Connor, and Phillip D. Tomporowski, *Exercise Psychology*, 2nd ed. (Champaign, IL: Human Kinetics, 2013).

11. Wolfram Schultz, "Reward Signaling by Dopamine Neurons," *The Neuroscientist* 7, no. 4 (2001): 293–302, DOI:10.1177/107385840100700406.

12. Mark Hamer and Costas I. Karageorghis, "Psychobiological Mechanisms of Exercise Dependence," *Sports Medicine* 37, no. 6 (2007): 477–84, DOI:10.2165/00007256-200737060-00002.

13. Malvin Janal, Edward W. D. Colt, W. Crawford Clark, and Murray Glusman, "Pain Sensitivity, Mood and Plasma Endocrine Levels Following Long-distance Running: Effects of Naloxone," *Pain* 19, no. 1 (1984): 13–25, DOI:10.1016/0304-3959(84)90061-7.

14. Arne Dietrich and William F. McDaniel, "Endocannabinoids and Exercise," *British Journal of Sports Medicine* 38, no. 5 (2004): 536–41, DOI:10.1136/bjsm.2004.011718.

15. Allan H. Goldfarb and Athanasios Z. Jamurtas, "Beta-endorphin Response to Exercise: An Update," *Sports Medicine* 24, no. 1 (1997): 8–16, DOI:10.2165/00007256-199724010-00002.

16. Lothar Schwarz and Wilfried Kindermann, "Changes in β-Endorphin Levels in Response to Aerobic and Anaerobic Exercise," *Sports Medicine* 13, no. 1 (1992): 25–36, DOI:10.2165/00007256-199213010-00003.

17. Lothar Schwarz and Wilfried Kindermann, "Beta-endorphin, Adrenocorticotropic Hormone, Cortisol and Catecholamines during Aerobic and Anaerobic Exercise," *European Journal of Applied Physiology* 61, nos. 3–4 (1990): 165–71, DOI:10.1007/BF00357593.

18. Helen C. Beh, Sarah Mathers, and John Holden, "EEG Correlates of Exercise Dependency," *International Journal of Psychophysiology* 23, nos. 1–2 (1996): 121–28, DOI:10.1016/0167-8760(96)00039-6.

19. Bruce E. Wexler, Christopher H. Gottschalk, Robert K. Fulbright, Isak Prohovnik, Cheryl M. Lacadie, Bruce J. Rounsaville, and John C. Gore, "Functional Magnetic Resonance Imaging of Cocaine Craving," *The American Journal of Psychiatry* 158, no. 1 (2001): 86–95, DOI:10.1176/appi.ajp.158.1.86.

20. Durand F. Jacobs, "A General Theory of Addictions: A New Theoretical Model," *Journal of Gambling Behavior* 2, no. 1 (1986): 15–31.

21. Attila Szabó, "Physical Activity and Psychological Dysfunction," in *Physical Activity and Psychological Well-being*, ed. Stuart J. H. Biddle, Ken Fox, and Steve Boutcher (New York: Routledge, 2000), 130–53.

22. Claire Carrier, "Addiction to Muscular Exercise: The Limit of Somatopsychology When Linked to Sport," *Addictions et travail* VST, no. 98 (2008): 35–41.

23. Alayne Yates, *Compulsive Exercise and the Eating Disorders* (New York: Brunner/Mazel, 1991).

24. Alayne Yates, *Compulsive Exercise and the Eating Disorders* (New York: Brunner/Mazel, 1991).

25. George E. Barnes, Robert P. Murray, David Patton, Peter M. Bentler, and Robert E. Anderson, *The Addiction-prone Personality* (New York: Kluwer Academic/Plenum Publishers, 2000).

26. Eric D. Martin and Kenneth J. Sher, "Family History of Alcoholism, Alcohol Use Disorders and the Five-factor Model of Personality," *Journal of Studies on Alcohol* 55, no. 1 (1994): 81–90.

27. Dean G. Kilpatrick, Deborah A. McAlhany, R. Layton McCurdy, Darlene Shaw, and John C. Roitzsch, "Aging, Alcoholism, Anxiety, and Sensation Seeking: An Exploratory Investigation," *Addictive Behavior* 7, no. 1 (1982): 97–100, DOI:10.1016/0306-4603(82)90033-8.

28. Ruben D. Baler and Nora D. Volkow, "Drug Addiction: The Neurobiology of Disrupted Self-control," *Trends in Molecular Medicine* 12, no. 12 (2006): 559–66, DOI:10.1016/j.molmed.2006.10.005.

29. Donald J. Samuels and Muriel Samuels, "Low Self-concept as a Cause of Drug Abuse," *Journal of Drug Education* 4, no. 4 (1974): 421–38, DOI:10.2190/VJHU-MRAR-NLG6-1XBH.

30. David S. Janowsky, Liyi Hong, Shirley Morter, and Laura Howe, "Underlying Personality Differences between Alcohol/Substance-use Disorder Patients with and without an Affective Disorder," *Alcohol & Alcoholism* 34, no. 3 (1999): 370–77, DOI:10.1093/alcalc/34.3.370.

31. Nathan Rosenberg, "MMPI Alcoholism Scales," *Journal of Clinical Psychology* 28, no. 4 (1972): 515–22, DOI:10.1002/1097-4679(197210)28:4&#60515::AID-JCLP2270280421&#623.0.CO;2-N.

32. Heather A. Hausenblas and Peter Giacobbi, "Relationship between Exercise Dependence Symptoms and Personality," *Personality and Individual Differences* 36, no. 6 (2004): 1265–73, DOI:10.1016/S0191-8869(03)00214-9.

33. Heather A. Hausenblas and Peter Giacobbi, "Relationship between Exercise Dependence Symptoms and Personality," *Personality and Individual Differences* 36, no. 6 (2004): 1265–73, DOI:10.1016/S0191-8869(03)00214-9.

34. Craig MacAndrew, "Male Alcoholics, Secondary Psychopathy and Eysenck's Theory of Personality," *Personality and Individual Differences* 1, no. 2 (1980): 151–60, DOI:10.1016/0191-8869(80)90033-1.

35. Paul T. Costa and Robert R. McCrae, *Revised NEO Personality Inventory (NEO-PI-R) and NEO Five-factor Inventory (NEO-FFI) Professional Manual* (Odessa, FL: Psychological Assessment Resources, 1992).

36. Mia Beck Lichtenstein, Erik Christiansen, Ask Elklit, Niels Bilenberg, and René Klinky Støving, "Exercise Addiction: A Study of Eating Disorder Symptoms, Quality of Life, Personality Traits and Attachment Styles," *Psychiatry Research* 215, no. 2 (2014): 410–16, DOI:10.1016/j.psychres.2013.11.010.

37. Centers for Disease Control and Prevention, "Healthy Weight—It's Not a Diet, It's a Lifestyle!" www.cdc.gov/healthyweight/assessing/bmi/adult_bmi/ (accessed February 22, 2014).

38. Alayne Yates, *Compulsive Exercise and the Eating Disorders* (New York: Brunner/Mazel, 1991).

39. Marilyn Freimuth, Sandy Moniz, and Shari R. Kim, "Clarifying Exercise Addiction: Differential Diagnosis, Co-occurring Disorders, and Phases of Addiction," *International Journal of Environmental Research and Public Health* 8, no. 10 (2011): 4069–81, DOI:10.3390/ijerph8104069.

40. David E. Smith, "Editor's Note: The Process Addictions and the New ASAM Definition of Addiction," *Journal of Psychoactive Drugs* 44, no. 1 (2012): 1–4, DOI:10.1080/02791072.2012.662105.

41. Krisztina Berczik, Attila Szabó, Mark D. Griffiths, Tamás Kurimay, Bernadette Kun, Róbert Urbán, and Zsolt Demetrovics, "Exercise Addiction: Symptoms, Diagnosis, Epidemiology, and Etiology," *Substance Use & Misuse* 47, no. 4 (2012): 403–17, DOI:10.3109/10826084.2011.639120.

42. Eugene V. Aidman and Simon Woollard, "The Influence of Self-reported Exercise Addiction on Acute Emotional and Physiological Responses to Brief Exercise Deprivation," *Psychology of Sport and Exercise* 4, no. 3 (2003): 225–36, DOI:10.1016/S1469-0292(02)00003-1.

43. American Society of Addiction Medicine, "Public Policy Statement: Definition of Addiction," www.asam.org/for-the-public/definition-of-addiction (accessed February 22, 2014).

44. Diane J. Bamber, Ian M. Cockerill, S. Rodgers, and Doug Carroll, "Diagnostic Criteria for Exercise Dependence in Women," *British Journal of Sports Medicine* 37, no. 5 (2003): 393–400, DOI:10.1136/bjsm.37.5.393.

5. WHAT IT DOES

1. Deborah A. Burton, Keith Stokes, and George M. Hall, "Physiological Effects of Exercise," *Continuing Education in Anaesthesia, Critical Care & Pain* 4, no. 6 (2004): 185–88, DOI:10.1093/bjaceaccp/mkh050.

2. Phillip A. Bishop, Eric Jones, and Krista A. Woods, "Recovery from Training: A Brief Review," *Journal of Strength & Conditioning Research* 22, no. 3 (2008): 1015–24, DOI:10.1519/JSC.0b013e31816eb518.

3. American Orthopaedic Society for Sports Medicine, "Overuse Injuries," www.sportsmed.org/uploadedFiles/Content/Patient/Sports_Tips/ ST%20Overuse%20Injuries%2008.pdf.

4. Els Clays, Dirk De Bacquer, Heidi Janssens, Bart De Clercq, Annalisa Casini, Lutgart Braeckman, France Kittel, Guy De Backer, and Andreas Holtermann, "The Association between Leisure Time Physical Activity and Coronary Heart Disease among Men with Different Work Demands: A Prospective Cohort Study," *European Journal of Epidemiology* 28, no. 3 (2013): 241–47, DOI:10.1007/s10654-013-9764-4.

5. Mathew Wilson, Rory O'Hanlon, Satyendra K. Prasad, A. Deighan, Peter D. Macmillan, Dave Oxborough, Richard Godfrey, Gillian Smith, Alicia Maceira, Sanjay Sharma, Keith P. George, and Gregory P. White, "Diverse Patterns of Myocardial Fibrosis in Lifelong, Veteran Endurance Athletes," *Journal of Applied Physiology* 110, no. 6 (2011): 1622–26.

6. Dominique Lecomte, Paul Fornes, Pierre Fouret, and Guy Nicolas, "Isolated Myocardial Fibrosis as a Cause of Sudden Cardiac Death and Its

Possible Relation to Myocarditis," *Journal of Forensic Sciences* 38, no. 3 (1993): 617–21.

7. Duck-chul Lee, Russell R. Pate, Carl J. Lavie, and Steven N. Blair, "Running and All-cause Mortality Risk: Is More Better?" ACSM Annual Meeting: World Congress on Exercise in Medicine, May 29–June 2, 2012, San Francisco, California.

8. Mary N. Sheppard, "The Fittest Person in the Morgue?" *Histopathology* 60, no. 3 (2012): 381–96, DOI:10.1111/j.1365-2559.2011.03852.x.

9. Jonathan H. Kim, Rajeev Malhotra, George Chiampas, Pierre d'Hemecourt, Chris Troyanos, John Cianca, Rex N. Smith, Thomas J. Wang, William O. Roberts, Paul D. Thompson, and Aaron L. Baggish, "Cardiac Arrest during Long-distance Running Races," *The New England Journal of Medicine* 366, no. 2 (2012): 130–40, DOI:10.1056/NEJMoa1106468.

10. Andreas P. Michaelides, Dimitris Soulis, Charalambos Antoniades, Alexios S. Antonopoulous, Antigoni Miliou, Nikolaos Ioakeimidis, Evangelos I. Chatzistamatiou, Constantinos Bakogiannis, Kyriakoula Marinou, Charalampos I. Liakos, and Christodoulos Stefanadis, "Exercise Duration as a Determinant of Vascular Function and Antioxidant Balance in Patients with Coronary Artery Disease," *Heart* 97, no. 10 (2011): 832–37, DOI:10.1136/hrt.2010.209080.

11. Charalambos Vlachopoulos, Despina Kardara, Aris Anastasakis, Katerina Baou, Dimitrios Terentes-Printzios, Dimitris Tousoulis, and Christodoulos Stefanadis, "Arterial Stiffness and Wave Reflections in Marathon Runners," *American Journal of Hypertension* 23, no. 9 (2010): 974–79, DOI: 10.1038/ajh.2010.99.

12. Barry J. Maron and Antonio Pelliccia, "The Heart of Trained Athletes: Cardiac Remodeling and the Risk of Sports, Including Sudden Death," *Circulation* 114, no. 15 (2006): 1633–44, DOI:10.1161/CIRCULATIONA-HA.106.613562.

13. Babette M. Pluim, Aeilko H. Zwinderman, Arnoud van der Laarse, and Ernst E. van der Wall, "The Athlete's Heart: A Meta-analysis of Cardiac Structure and Function," *Circulation* 101, no. 3 (2000): 336–44, DOI:10.1161/01.CIR.101.3.336.

14. Jonathan G. Schwartz, Stacia Merkel-Kraus, Sue Duval, Kevin Harris, Gretchen Peichel, John R. Lesser, Thomas Knickelbine, Bjorn Flygenring, Terry R. Longe, Catherine Pastorius, William R. Roberts, Stephen C. Oesterle, and Robert S. Schwartz, "Does Elite Athleticism Enhance or Inhibit Coronary Artery Plaque Formation? A Prospective Multidetector CTA Study of Men Completing Marathons for at Least 25 Consecutive Years," paper presented at the American College of Cardiology 2010 Scientific Session, Atlanta, GA (2010): 1271–330, www.abstractsonline.com/Plan/ViewAbstract.aspx?mID=2444&sKey=747bc0a9-d52f-4671-a6c7-e189fbc76e0a&

cKey=8d57d453-a124-4c89-a1d0-da559dbfa754&mKey=7a9907ef-0b49-4421-a7ae-7e7f1ebb9402 (accessed March 12, 2014).

15. Antonio Pelliccia, Barry J. Maron, Fernando M. Di Paolo, Alessandro Biffi, Filippo M. Quattrini, Cataldo Pisicchio, Alessangra Roselli, Stefano Caselli, and Franco Culasso, "Prevalence and Clinical Significance of Left Atrial Remodeling in Competitive Athletes," *Journal of the American College of Cardiology* 46, no. 4 (2005): 690–96, DOI:10.1016/j.jacc.2005.04.052.

16. Barry J. Maron, "Hypertrophic Cardiomyopathy: A Systematic Review," *The Journal of the American Medical Association: Clinical Cardiology* 287, no. 10 (2002): 1308–20, DOI:10.1001/jama.287.10.1308.

17. Antonio Pelliccia, Barry J. Maron, Antonio Spataro, Michael A. Proschan, and Paolo Spirito, "The Upper Limit of Physiologic Cardiac Hypertrophy in Highly Trained Elite Athletes," *The New England Journal of Medicine* 324, no. 5 (1991): 295–301, DOI:10.1056/NEJM199101313240504.

18. Christopher Uebleis, Alexander Becker, Ines Griesshammer, Paul Cumming, Christoph Becker, Michael Schmidt, Peter Bartenstein, and Marcus Hacker, "Stable Coronary Artery Disease: Prognostic Value of Myocardial Perfusion SPECT in Relation to Coronary Calcium Scoring—Long-term Follow-up," *Radiology* 252, no. 3 (2009): 682–90, DOI:10.1148/radiol.2531082137.

19. Priscilla M. Clarkson, "Exertional Rhabdomyolysis and Acute Renal Failure in Marathon Runners," *Sports Medicine* 37 nos. 4–5 (2007): 361–63, DOI:10.2165/00007256-200737040-00022.

20. Peter A. McCullough, Kavitha M. Chinnaiyan, Michael J. Gallagher, James M. Colar, Timothy Geddes, Jeffrey M. Gold, and Justin E. Trivax, "Changes in Renal Markers and Acute Kidney Injury after Marathon Running," *Nephrology* 16, no. 2 (2011): 194–99, www.ncbi.nlm.nih.gov/pubmed/21272132.

21. Raymond Vanholder, Mehmet Sükrü Sever, Ekrem Erek, and Norbert Lameire, "Rhabdomyolysis," *Journal of the American Society of Nephrology* 11, no. 8 (2000): 1553–61.

22. L. S. Baylor and Anthony C. Hackney, "Resting Thyroid and Leptin Hormone Changes in Women Following Intense, Prolonged Exercise Training," *European Journal of Applied Physiology* 88, nos. 4–5 (2003): 480–84.

23. Thomas W. Boyden, Richard W. Pamenter, Thomas C. Rotkis, Philip Stanforth, and Jack H. Wilmore, "Thyroidal Changes Associated with Endurance Training in Women," *Medicine & Science in Sports & Exercise* 16, no. 3 (1984): 234–46.

24. A.D.A.M. Medical Encyclopedia, "Metabolic Acidosis," PubMed Health, www.ncbi.nlm.nih.gov/pubmedhealth/PMH0001376.

25. Gary Kamen, *Foundations of Exercise Science* (Philadelphia: Lippincott Williams & Wilkins, 2001), 21.

26. Mary B. Johnson and Steven M. Thiese, "A Review of Overtraining Syndrome—Recognizing the Signs and Symptoms," *Journal of Athletic Training* 27, no. 4 (1992): 352–54.

27. George N. Wade and Juli E. Jones, "Neuroendocrinology of Nutritional Infertility," *American Journal of Physiology: Regulatory, Integrative and Comparative Physiology* 287, no. 6 (2004): R1277–96, www.ncbi.nlm.nih.gov/pubmed/15528398.

28. American College of Sports Medicine, "The Female Athlete Triad," www.acsm.org/docs/brochures/the-female-athlete-triad.pdf.

29. Linnea R. Goodman and Michelle P. Warren, "The Female Athlete and Menstrual Function," *Current Opinion in Obstetrics and Gynecology* 17, no. 15 (2005): 446–70.

30. Aurelia Nattiv, Anne B. Loucks, Melinda M. Manore, Charlotte F. Sanborn, Jorunn Sundgot-Borgen, and Michelle P. Warren, "American College of Sports Medicine Position Stand: The Female Athlete Triad," *Medicine and Science in Sports and Exercise* 39, no. 10 (2007): 1867–82.

31. Jill Thein-Nissenbaum, "Long Term Consequences of the Female Athlete Triad," *Maturitas* 75, no. 2 (2013): 107–12.

32. Karen Hind, "Recovery of Bone Mineral Density and Fertility in a Former Amenorrheic Athlete," *Journal of Sports Science & Medicine* 7, no. 3 (2008): 415–18.

33. Anne Loucks, "Refutation of 'the Myth of the Female Athlete Triad,'" *British Journal of Sports Medicine* 41, no. 1 (2007): 55–57.

34. Mona M. Shangold and H. S. Levine, "The Effect of Marathon Training upon Menstrual Function," *American Journal of Obstetrics and Gynecology* 143, no. 8 (1982): 862–69.

35. Herman Adlercreutz, Mikko Härkönen, Kimmo Kuoppasalmi, Hannu Näveri, Ilpo Huhtaniemi, Heiki O. Tikkanen, Kari Remes, Adriano Dessypris, and Jukka Karvonen, "Effect of Training on Plasma Anabolic and Catabolic Steroid Hormones and Their Response during Physical Exercise," *International Journal of Sports Medicine* 7, suppl. no. 1 (1986): 27–28, DOI:10.1055/s-2008-1025798.

36. William E. Buckley, Charles E. Yesalis III, Karl E. Friedi, William A. Anderson, Andrea L. Streit, and James E. Wright, "Estimated Prevalence of Anabolic Steroid Use among Male High School Seniors," *The Journal of the American Medical Association* 260, no. 23 (1988): 3441–45, DOI:10.1001/jama.1988.03410230059028.

37. Graham Bolding, Lorraine Sherr, and Jonathan Elford, "Use of Anabolic Steroids and Associated Health Risks among Gay Men Attending London Gyms," *Addiction* 97, no. 2 (2002): 195–203, DOI:10.1046/j.1360-0442.2002.00031.x.

38. Mary B. Johnson and Steven M. Thiese, "A Review of Overtraining Syndrome—Recognizing the Signs and Symptoms," *Journal of Athletic Training* 27, no. 4 (1992): 352–54.

39. Gretchen Reynolds, "Crash and Burnout," *New York Times*, www.nytimes.com/2008/03/02/sports/playmagazine/02play-physed.html?pagewanted=all.

40. Sean O. Richardson, Mark B. Andersen, and Tony Morris, *Overtraining Athletes* (Champaign, IL: Human Kinetics, 2008), 16–17.

41. Sue L. Hooper, Laurel Traeger Mackinnon, Richard D. Gordon, and Anthony W. Bachmann, "Hormonal Responses of Elite Swimmers to Overtraining," *Medicine and Science in Sports and Exercise* 25, no. 6 (1993): 741–47.

42. William P. Morgan, Patrick J. O'Connor, Phillip B. Sparling, and Russ R. Pate, "Psychological Characterizations of the Elite Female Distance Runner," *International Journal of Sports Medicine* 8, suppl. no. 2 (1987): 124–31.

43. Donald C. McKenzie, "Markers of Excessive Exercise," *Canadian Journal of Applied Physiology* 24, no. 1 (1999): 66–73.

44. Marilyn Freimuth, Sandy Moniz, and Shari R. Kim, "Clarifying Exercise Addiction: Differential Diagnosis, Co-occurring Disorders, and Phases of Addiction," *International Journal of Environmental Research and Public Health*, 8, no. 10 (2011): 4069–81, DOI:10.3390/ijerph8104069.

45. Krisztina Berczik, Attila Szabó, Mark D. Griffiths, Tamás Kurimay, Bernadette Kun, Róbert Urbán, and Zsolt Demetrovics, "Exercise Addiction: Symptoms, Diagnosis, Epidemiology, and Etiology," *Substance Use & Misuse* 47, no. 4 (2012): 403–17, DOI:10.3109/10826084.2011.639120.

46. Andrew Baum and Donna M. Polsusnzy, "Health Psychology: Mapping Biobehavioral Contributions to Health and Illness," *Annual Review of Psychology* 50 (1999): 137–63, DOI:10.1146/annurev.psych.50.1.137.

6. WHY IT HAPPENS

1. Jennifer Ashton, "Addicted to Exercise," Health and Wellness, CBS News, November 2, 2009, www.cbsnews.com/videos/addicted-to-exercise (accessed April 2, 2014).

2. Floyd Henry Allport, "The J-curve Hypothesis of Conforming Behavior," *Journal of Social Psychology* 5 (1934): 141–83.

3. Fitspoholic, Daily Motivation, http://fitspoholic.tumblr.com/tagged/fitspoholic (accessed March 25, 2014).

4. Kevin Moore, "The Six Most Shockingly Irresponsible 'Fitspiration' Photos," REEMBODY, http://reembody.me/2013/09/10/the-6-most-shockingly-irresponsible-fitspiration-photos (accessed March 25, 2014).

5. Fitspoholic Daily Motivation, http://fitspoholic.tumblr.com/tagged/fitspoholic (accessed March 25, 2014).

6. Fitspoholic Daily Motivation, http://fitspoholic.tumblr.com/tagged/fitspoholic (accessed March 25, 2014).

7. Kelly D. Brownell, "Dieting and the Search for the Perfect Body: Where Physiology and Culture Collide," *Behavior Therapy* 22, no. 1 (1991): 1–12, DOI:10.1016/S0005-7894(05)80239-4.

8. Morris Rosenberg and Leonard I. Pearlin, "Social Class and Self-esteem among Children and Adults," *American Journal of Sociology* 84, no. 1 (1978): 53–77.

9. Nicholas Emler, *Self-esteem: The Costs and Causes of Low Self-worth* (York, UK: Joseph Rowntree Foundation, 2001).

10. Nicholas Emler, *Self-Esteem: The Costs and Causes of Low Self-worth* (York, UK: Joseph Rowntree Foundation, 2001).

11. Richard M. Lerner, Stuart A. Karabenick, and Joyce L. Stuart, "Relations among Physical Attractiveness, Body Attitudes, and Self-concept in Male and Female College Students," *The Journal of Psychology: Interdisciplinary and Applied* 85, no. 1 (1973): 119–29, DOI:10.1080/00223980.1973.9923870.

12. Caroline Davis and Michael Cowles, "Body Image and Exercise: A Study of Relationships and Comparisons between Physically Active Men and Women," *Sex Roles* 25, nos. 1–2 (1991): 33–44, DOI:10.1007/BF00289315.

13. Adrian Furnham, Nicola Badmin, and Ian Sneade, "Body Image Dissatisfaction: Gender Differences in Eating Attitudes, Self-esteem, and Reasons for Exercise," *The Journal of Psychology* 13, no. 6 (2002): 581–96.

14. Joanne V. Wood, W. Q. Elaine Perunovic, and John W. Lee, "Positive Self-statements: Power for Some, Peril for Others," *Psychological Science* 20, no. 7 (2009): 860–66, DOI:10.1111/j.1467-9280.2009.02370.x.

15. Heather Hausenblas and Elizabeth A. Fallon, "Exercise and Body Image: A Meta-analysis," *Psychology & Health* 21, no. 1 (2006): 33–47, DOI:10.1080/14768320500105270.

16. Heather Hausenblas, Britton W. Brewer, and Judy L. Van Raalte, "Self-presentation and Exercise," *Journal of Applied Sport Psychology* 16, no. 1 (2004): 3–18, DOI:10.1080/10413200490260026.

17. Jennifer Crocker, "The Costs of Seeking Self-esteem," *Journal of Social Issues* 58, no. 3 (2002): 597–615.

18. Jennifer Crocker, "The Costs of Seeking Self-esteem," *Journal of Social Issues* 58, no. 3 (2002): 597–615.

19. Jennifer Crocker, "The Costs of Seeking Self-esteem," *Journal of Social Issues* 58, no. 3 (2002): 597–615.

20. Edward L. Deci and Richard M. Ryan, "Human Autonomy: The Basis for True Self-esteem," in *Efficacy, Agency, and Self-esteem*, ed. Michael H. Kernis (New York: Plenum, 1995), 31–49.

21. Kristen Neff, *Self-compassion* (New York: HarperCollins, 2011).

22. Jennifer Crocker, "The Costs of Seeking Self-esteem," *Journal of Social Issues* 58, no. 3 (2002): 597–615.

23. Magnus Lindwall and Kathleen A. Martin Ginis, "Moving towards a Favorable Image: The Self-presentational Benefits of Exercise and Physical Activity," *Scandinavian Journal of Psychology* 47, no. 3 (2006): 209–17.

24. Alayne Yates, *Compulsive Exercise and the Eating Disorders* (New York: Brunner/Mazel, 1991).

25. Alayne Yates, *Compulsive Exercise and the Eating Disorders* (New York: Brunner/Mazel, 1991).

26. Alayne Yates, *Compulsive Exercise and the Eating Disorders* (New York: Brunner/Mazel, 1991).

27. Alayne Yates, *Compulsive Exercise and the Eating Disorders* (New York: Brunner/Mazel, 1991).

28. Centers for Disease Control and Prevention, "Participation in Leisure-time Aerobic and Muscle-strengthening Activities That Meet the Federal 2008 Physical Activity Guidelines for Americans among Adults Aged 18 and over, by Selected Characteristics: United States, Selected Years 1998–2012," www.cdc.gov/nchs/data/hus/2012/067.pdf (accessed March 28, 2014).

29. American College of Sports Medicine, "Research Yields Fitness Motivation Tips for a Healthy New Year," www.acsm.org/about-acsm/media-room/news-releases/2011/08/01/research-yields-fitness-motivation-tips-for-a-healthy-new-year (accessed March 25, 2014).

30. U.S. Department of Health and Human Services, "Physical Activity Guidelines for Americans," www.health.gov/paguidelines/guidelines/chapter6.aspx (accessed March 26, 2014).

31. Centers for Disease Control and Prevention, "National Hospital Ambulatory Medical Care Survey: 2010 Emergency Department Summary Tables," www.cdc.gov/nchs/data/ahcd/nhamcs_emergency/2010_ed_web_tables.pdf (accessed March 26, 2014).

32. Nolan Caldwell, Tanja Srebotnjak, Tiffany Wang, and Renee Hsia, "'How Much Will I Get Charged for This?' Patient Charges for Top Ten Diagnoses in the Emergency Department," *PLOSone* 8, no. 1 (2013): e55491, DOI:10.1371/journal.pone.0055491.

33. Melissa Dahl, "Gym-goers Trip, Flip, and Fall in Pursuit of Fitness," NBCNews.com, www.nbcnews.com/id/35127528/ns/health-fitness/t/gym-goers-trip-flip-fall-pursuit-fitness (accessed March 26, 2014).

34. American Association of Neurological Surgeons, "Sports-related Head Injury," www.aans.org/Patient Information/Conditions and Treatments/Sports-Related Head Injury.aspx (accessed March 26, 2014).

35. National Association of Anorexia Nervosa, "General Information about Eating Disorders," www.anad.org/get-information/about-eating-disorders/general-information (accessed March 26, 2014).

36. Marilyn Freimuth, Sandy Moniz, and Shari R. Kim, "Clarifying Exercise Addiction: Differential Diagnosis, Co-occurring Disorders, and Phases of Addiction," *International Journal of Environmental Research and Public Health* 8, no. 10 (2011): 4069–81, DOI:10.3390/ijerph8104069.

37. Yafu Zhao and William Encinos, "Hospitalizations for Eating Disorders from 1999 to 2006," Statistical Brief #70, *Healthcare Cost and Utilization Project (HCUP)* (Rockville, MD: Agency for Healthcare Research and Quality, January 2011), www.hcup-us.ahrq.gov/reports/statbriefs/sb70.jsp.

38. Judith M. Conn, Joseph L. Annest, and Julie Gilchrist, "Sports and Recreation Related Injury Episodes in the U.S. Population, 1997–99," *Injury Prevention* 9, no. 2 (2003): 117–23, DOI:10.1136/ip.9.2.117.

39. Zachary Y. Kerr, Christy L. Collins, and R. Dawn Comstock, "Epidemiology of Weight Training–related Injuries Presenting to United States Emergency Departments," *The American Journal of Medicine* 38, no. 4 (2010): 765–71, DOI:10.1177/0363546509351560.

40. Astrid Bovens, Geert Janssen, H. G. W. Vermeer, Jean H. Hoeberigs, Marie P. Janssen, Frans T. J. Verstappen, "Occurrence of Running Injuries in Adults Following a Supervised Training Program," *International Journal of Sports Medicine* 10, no. S3 (1989): S186–S190, DOI:10.1055/s-2007-1024970.

41. Jennifer M. Hootman, Carol A. Macera, Barbara E. Ainsworth, Malissa Martin, Cheryl L. Addy, and Steven N. Blair, "Association among Physical Activity Level, Cardiorespiratory Fitness, and Risk of Musculoskeletal Injury," *American Journal of Epidemiology* 154, no. 3 (2001): 251–58, DOI:10.1093/aje/154.3.251.

42. Julie Gilchrist, Karen E. Thomas, Likang Xu, Lisa C. McGuire, and Victor Coronado, "Nonfatal Sports and Recreation Related Traumatic Brain Injuries among Children and Adolescents Treated in Emergency Departments in the United States, 2001–2009," *Morbidity and Mortality Weekly Report* 60, no. 39 (2011): 1337–42.

43. Jean A. Langlois, Wesley Rutland-Brown, and Marlena M. Wald, "The Epidemiology and Impact of Traumatic Brain Injury: A Brief Overview," *Journal of Head Trauma Rehabilitation* 21, no. 5 (2006): 375–78.

44. Emmett Jones, "Athletic Apparel Revenue to Reach $180 Billion a Year by 2018," *Sports Business Digest,* http://sportsbusinessdigest.com/2013/03/athletic-apparel-revenue-to-reach-180-billion-a-year-by-2018 (accessed March 26, 2014).

8. WHAT TO DO ABOUT IT

1. Heather A. Hausenblas, Brian J. Cook, and Nickles I. Chittester, "Can Exercise Treat Eating Disorders?" *Exercise and Sport Sciences Reviews* 36, no. 1 (2008): 43–47.

2. Louisa W. Ng, Daniel P. Ng, and Wai P. Wong, "Is Supervised Exercise Training Safe in Patients with Anorexia Nervosa? A Meta-analysis," *Physiotherapy* 99, no. 1 (2013): 1–11, DOI:10.1016/j.physio.2012.05.006.

3. James O. Prochaska and Wayne F. Velicer, "The Transtheoretical Model of Health Behavior Change," *American Journal of Health Promotion* 12, no. 1 (1997): 38–48.

4. Sarah J. Cockell, Josie Geller, and Wolfgang Linden, "Decisional Balance in Anorexia Nervosa: Capitalizing on Ambivalence," *European Eating Disorders Review* 11, no. 2 (2003): 75–89.

5. Cynthia M. Bulik and Nancy D. Berkman, "Eating Disorders: Newer Practice Guidelines Reinforce Severity of Conditions but Still Reflect Deficits in Knowledge Base," National Guideline Clearinghouse, February 25, 2008, www.guideline.gov/expert/printView.aspx?id=16450 (accessed March 17, 2014).

6. Kate B. Wolitzky-Taylor, Joanna J. Arch, David Rosenfield, and Michelle G. Craske, "Moderators and Non-specific Predictors of Treatment Outcome for Anxiety Disorders: A Comparison of Cognitive Behavioral Therapy to Acceptance and Commitment Therapy," *Journal of Consulting and Clinical Psychology* 80, no. 5 (2012): 786–99, DOI:10.1037/a0029418.

7. Kathryn McHugh, Bridget A. Hearon, and Michael W. Otto, "Cognitive-behavioral Therapy for Substance Use Disorders," *Psychiatric Clinics of North America* 33, no. 3 (2010): 511–25.

8. Reef Karim and Priya Chaudhri, "Behavioral Addictions: An Overview," *Journal of Psychoactive Drugs* 44, no. 1 (2012): 5–17, DOI:10.1080/02791072.2012.662859.

9. Jeffrey A. Cully and Andra L. Teten, *A Therapist's Guide to Brief Cognitive Behavioral Therapy* (Houston, TX: Department of Veterans Affairs South Central MIRECC, 2008).

10. Marco Di Nicola, Giovanni Martinotti, Marianna Mazza, Daniela Tedeschi, Gino Pozzi, and Luigi Janiri, "Quetiapine as Add-on Treatment for

Bipolar I Disorder with Comorbid Compulsive Buying and Physical Exercise Addiction," *Progress in Neuro-psychopharmacology & Biological Psychiatry* 34, no. 4 (2010): 713–14, DOI:10.1016/j.pnpbp.2010.03.013.

11. Kiranmai Gorla and Maju Mathews, "Pharmacological Treatment of Eating Disorders," *Psychiatry* 2, no. 6 (2005): 42–48.

12. J. Michael Bostwick, "Internet Sex Addiction Treated with Naltrexone," *Mayo Clinic Proceedings* 83, no. 2 (2008): 226–30.

13. James M. Smoliga, Joseph A. Baur, and Heather A. Hausenblas, "Resveratrol and Health: A Comprehensive Review of Human Clinical Studies," *Molecular Nutrition and Food Research* 55, no. 8 (2011): 1129–41, DOI:10.1002/mnfr.201100143.

14. Tina-Tinkara Peternelj and Jeff S. Coombes, "Antioxidant Supplementation during Exercise Training: Beneficial or Detrimental?" *Sports Medicine* 41, no. 12 (2011): 1043–69, DOI:10.2165/11594400-000000000-00000.

15. Heather A. Hausenblas, Debbie Saha, Pamela Jean Dubyak, and Stephen Douglas Anton, "Saffron (*Crocus Sativus L.*) and Major Depressive Disorder: A Meta-analysis of Randomized Clinical Trials," *Journal of Integrative Medicine* 11, no. 6 (2013): 377–83, DOI:10.3736/jintegrmed2013056.

16. Robert D. Zettle, "The Evolution of a Contextual Approach to Therapy: From Comprehensive Distancing to ACT," *International Journal of Behavioral Consultation and Therapy* 1, no. 2 (2005): 77–89.

17. Katie Sharp, "A Review of Acceptance and Commitment Therapy with Anxiety Disorders," *International Journal of Psychology & Psychological Therapy* 12, no. 3 (2012): 359–72.

18. Adrienne S. Juarascio, Evan M. Forman, and James D. Herbert, "Acceptance and Commitment Therapy versus Cognitive Therapy for the Treatment of Comorbid Eating Pathology," *Behavior Modification* 34, no. 2 (2010): 175–90.

19. Francisco J. Ruiz, "Acceptance and Commitment Therapy versus Traditional Cognitive Behavioral Therapy: A Systematic Review and Meta-analysis of Current Empirical Evidence," *International Journal of Psychology & Psychological Therapy* 12, no. 2 (2012): 333–57.

20. Jean L. Kristeller, Ruth A. Baer, and Ruth Quillian-Wolever, "Mindfulness-based Approaches to Eating Disorders," in *Mindfulness-based Treatment Approaches: Clinician's Guide to Evidence Base and Applications*, ed. Ruth A. Baer (London: Elsevier, 2006), 75–91.

21. John D. Teasdale, Zindel V. Segal, J. Mark G. Williams, Valerie A. Ridgeway, Judith M. Soulsby, and Mark A. Lau, "Prevention of Relapse/Recurrence in Major Depression by Mindfulness-based Cognitive Therapy," *Journal of Consulting and Clinical Psychology* 68, no. 4 (2000): 615–23, DOI:10.1037/0022-006X.68.4.615.

22. Aleksandra Zglerska, David Rabago, Neharika Chawla, Kenneth Kushner, Robert Koehler, and Alan Marlatt, "Mindfulness Meditation for Substance Use Disorders: Systematic Review," *Substance Abuse* 30, no. 4 (2009): 266–94, DOI:10.1080/08897070903250019.

23. Paul Chadwick, Stephanie Hughes, Daphne Russell, Ian Russel, and Dave Dagnan, "Mindfulness Groups for Distressing Voices and Paranoia: A Replication and Randomized Feasibility Trial," *Behavioural and Cognitive Psychotherapy* 37, no. 4 (2009): 403–12, DOI:10.1017/S1352465809990166.

24. David Shannahoff-Khalsa, Laura E. Ray, Saul Levine, Christopher C. Gallen, Barb J. Schwartz, and John J. Sidorowich, "Randomized Controlled Trial of Yogic Meditation Techniques for Patients with Obsessive Compulsive Disorder," *CNS Spectrums* 4, no. 12 (1999): 34–47.

25. Graham Kirkwood, Hagen Rampes, Veronica Tuffrey, Janet Richardson, and Karen Pilkington, "Yoga for Anxiety: A Systematic Review of the Research Evidence," *British Journal of Sports Medicine* 39, no. 12 (2005): 884–91, DOI:10.1136/bjsm.2005.018069.

26. Roberto Olivardia, "Muscle Dysmorphia: Characteristics, Assessment, and Treatment," in *The Muscular Ideal: Psychological, Social and Medical Perspectives*, ed. J. Kevin Thompson and Guy Cafri (Washington, DC: American Psychological Association, 2007), 123–39.

27. Frederick G. Grieve, Natalie Truba, and Sandy Bowersox, "Etiology, Assessment, and Treatment of Muscle Dysmorphia," *Journal of Cognitive Psychotherapy* 23, no. 4 (2009): 306–14.

28. Kelly Hamilton and Gören Waller, "Media Influences on Body Size Estimation in Anorexia and Bulimia: An Experimental Study," *British Journal of Psychiatry* 162 (1993): 837–40.

29. Kelly P. Arbour and Kathleen A. Martin Ginnis, "Effects of Exposure of Muscular and Hypermuscular Images on Young Men's Muscularity Dissatisfaction and Body Dissatisfaction," *Body Image* 3, no. 2 (2006): 153–62, DOI:10.1016/j.bodyim.2006.03.004.

30. Sarah Grogan and Nicola Wainwright, "Growing Up in the Culture of Slenderness: Girls' Experiences of Body Dissatisfaction," *Women's Studies International Forum* 19, no. 6 (1996): 665–73, DOI:10.1016/S0277-5395(96)00076-3.

31. Jill A. Cattarin, Kevin Thompson, Carmen Thomas, and Robyn Williams, "Body Image, Mood, and Televised Images of Attractiveness: The Role of Social Comparison," *Journal of Social and Clinical Psychology* 19, no. 2 (2000): 220–39, DOI:10.1521/jscp.2000.19.2.220.

32. Janine M. Philips and Murray J. N. Drummond, "An Investigation into the Body Image Perception, Body Satisfaction and Exercise Expectations of

Male Fitness Leaders: Implications for Professional Practice," *Leisure Studies* 20, no. 2 (2001): 95–105.

33. Alayne Yates, *Compulsive Exercise and the Eating Disorders* (New York: Brunner/Mazel, 1991).

10. FREQUENTLY ASKED QUESTIONS

1. Eugene V. Aidman and Simon Woollard, "The Influence of Self-reported Exercise Addiction on Acute Emotional and Physiological Responses to Brief Exercise Deprivation," *Psychology of Sport and Exercise* 4, no. 3 (2003): 225–36, DOI:10.1016/S1469-0292(02)00003-1.

2. Patrick J. Carnes, Robert E. Murray, and Louis Charpentier, "Bargains with Chaos: Sex Addicts and Addiction Interaction Disorder," *Sexual Addiction and Compulsivity: The Journal of Treatment and Prevention* 12, nos. 2–3 (2005): 79–120, DOI:10.1080/10720160500201371.

3. Michel Lejoyeux, Marine Avril, Charlotte Richoux, Houcine Embouazza, and Fabrizia Nivoli, "Prevalence of Exercise Dependence and Other Behavioral Addictions among Clients of a Parisian Fitness Room," *Comprehensive Psychiatry* 49, no. 4 (2008): 353–58, DOI:10.1016/j.comppsych.2007.12.005.

4. Samantha A. Haylett, Geoffrey M. Stephenson, and Robert M. H. Le-Fever, "Covariation of Addictive Behaviors: A Study of Addictive Orientation Using the Shorter PROMIS Questionnaire," *Addictive Behaviors* 29, no. 1 (2004): 61–71, DOI:10.1016/S0306-4603(03)00083-2.

5. Vance V. MacLaren and Lisa A. Best, "Multiple Addictive Behaviors in Young Adults: Student Norms for the Shorter PROMIS Questionnaire," *Addictive Behaviors* 35, no. 3 (2010): 252–55, DOI:10.1016/j.addbeh.2009.09.023.

6. Alan J. George, "Central Nervous System Stimulants," *Best Practice & Research Clinical Endocrinology & Metabolism* 14, no. 1 (2000): 79–88, DOI:10.1053/beem.2000.0055.

7. National Institute on Drug Abuse, The Science of Drug Abuse and Addiction, "DrugFacts: Anabolic Steroids," www.drugabuse.gov/publications/drugfacts/anabolic-steroids (accessed February 22, 2014).

8. Heather A. Slay, Jumi Hayaki, Melissa A. Napolitano, and Kelly D. Brownell, "Motivations for Running and Eating Attitudes in Obligatory versus Nonobligatory Runners," *International Journal of Eating Disorders* 23, no. 3 (1998): 267–75, DOI:10.1002/(SICI)1098-108X(199804)23:3&#60267::AID-EAT4&#623.0.CO;2-H.

9. Aviv Weinstein and Yitzhak Weinstein, "Exercise Addiction—Diagnosis, Bio-psychological Mechanisms and Treatment Issues," *Current Pharmaceutical Design* 20 (2014): 1–8, DOI:10.2174/13816128113199990614.

10. Michel Lejoyeux, Marine Avril, Charlotte Richoux, Houcine Embouazza, and Fabrizia Nivoli, "Prevalence of Exercise Dependence and Other Behavioral Addictions among Clients of a Parisian Fitness Room," *Comprehensive Psychiatry* 49, no. 4 (2008): 353–58, DOI:10.1016/j.comppsych.2007.12.005.

11. Mark D. Griffiths, Attila Szabó, and Annabel Terry, "The Exercise Addiction Inventory: A Quick and Easy Screening Tool for Health Practitioners," *British Journal of Sports Medicine* 39, no. 6 (2005): 30–31.

12. Attila Szabó and Mark D. Griffiths, "Exercise Addiction in British Sport Science Students," *International Journal of Mental Health and Addiction* 5, no. 1 (2007): 25–28.

13. Claudia Ravaldi, Alfredo Vannacci, Teresa Zucchi, Edoardo Mannucci, Pier Luigi Cabras, Maura Boldrini, Loriana Murciano, Carlo Maria Rotella, and Valdo Ricca, "Eating Disorders and Body Image Disturbances among Ballet Dancers, Gymnasium Users and Body Builders," *Psychopathology* 36, no. 5 (2003): 247–54, DOI:10.1159/000073450.

14. Heather A. Hausenblas and Danielle Symons Downs, "Relationship among Sex, Imagery and Exercise Dependence Symptoms," *Psychology of Addictive Behaviors* 16, no. 2 (2002): 169–72, DOI:10.1037/0893-164X.16.2.169.

15. Krisztina Berczik, Attila Szabó, Mark D. Griffiths, Tamás Kurimay, Bernadette Kun, Róbert Urbán, and Zsolt Demetrovics, "Exercise Addiction: Symptoms, Diagnosis, Epidemiology, and Etiology," *Substance Use & Misuse* 47, no. 4 (2012): 403–17, DOI:10.3109/10826084.2011.639120.

16. Sebastiano Costa, Heather A. Hausenblas, Patrizia Oliva, Francesca Cuzzocrea, and Rosalba Larcan, "The Role of Age, Gender, Mood States and Exercise Frequency on Exercise Dependence," *Journal of Behavioral Addictions* 2, no. 4 (2013): 216–23, DOI:10.1556/JBA.2.2013.014.

17. Heather A. Hausenblas and Elizabeth A. Fallon, "Relationship among Body Image, Exercise Behavior, and Exercise Dependence Symptoms," *International Journal of Eating Disorders* 32, no. 2 (2002): 179–85, DOI:10.1002/eat.10071.

18. Randy O. Frost and Gail Steketee, "Perfectionism in Obsessive-compulsive Disorder Patients," *Behaviour Research and Therapy* 35, no. 4 (1997): 291–96, DOI:10.1016/S0005-7967(96)00108-8.

19. James H. O'Keefe and Carl J. Lavie, "Run for Your Life . . . at a Comfortable Speed and Not Too Far," *Heart* 99, no. 8 (2013): 516–19, DOI:10.1136/heartjnl-2012-302886.

20. James H. O'Keefe and Carl J. Lavie, "Run for Your Life . . . at a Comfortable Speed and Not Too Far," *Heart* 99, no. 8 (2013): 516–19, DOI:10.1136/heartjnl-2012-302886.

21. Sebastiano Costa, Heather A. Hausenblas, Patrizia Oliva, Francesca Cuzzocrea, and Rosalba Larcan, "The Role of Age, Gender, Mood States and Exercise Frequency on Exercise Dependence," *Journal of Behavioral Addictions* 2, no. 4 (2013): 216–23, DOI:10.1556/JBA.2.2013.014.

22. Kira S. Birditt, Karen L. Fingerman, and David M. Almeida, "Age Differences in Exposure and Reactions to Interpersonal Tensions: A Daily Diary Study," *Psychology and Aging* 20, no. 2 (2005): 330–40, DOI:10.1037/0882-7974.20.2.330.

23. Carol Magai, Nathan S. Consedine, Yulia S. Krivoshekova, Elizabeth Kudadje-Gyamfi, and Renee McPherson, "Emotion Experience and Expression across the Adult Life Span: Insights from a Multimodal Assessment Study," *Psychology and Aging* 21, no. 2 (2006): 303–17, DOI:10.1037/0882-7974.21.2.303.

24. Aviv Weinstein and Yitzhak Weinstein, "Exercise Addiction—Diagnosis, Bio-psychological Mechanisms and Treatment Issues," *Current Pharmaceutical Design* 20 (2014): 1–8, DOI:10.2174/13816128113199990614.

25. Michel Lejoyeux, Marine Avril, Charlotte Richoux, Houcine Embouazza, and Fabrizia Nivoli, "Prevalence of Exercise Dependence and Other Behavioral Addictions among Clients of a Parisian Fitness Room," *Comprehensive Psychiatry* 49, no. 4 (2008): 353–58, DOI:10.1016/j.comppsych.2007.12.005.

26. James H. O'Keefe and Carl J. Lavie, "Run for Your Life . . . at a Comfortable Speed and Not Too Far," *Heart* 99, no. 8 (2013): 516–19, DOI:10.1136/heartjnl-2012-302886.

27. Robin L. Line and George S. Rust, "Acute Exertional Rhabdomyolysis," *Family Physician* 52, no. 2 (1995): 502–6.

28. Christian Schmied and Mats Borjesson, "Sudden Cardiac Death in Athletes," *Journal of Internal Medicine* 275, no. 2 (2014): 93–103, DOI:10.1111/joim.12184.

29. Wendy Russell, "Yoga and Vertebral Arteries," *British Medical Journal* 1, no. 5801 (1972): 685.

30. Frederick S. Cohen and Judianne Densen-Gerber, "A Study of the Relationship between Child Abuse and Drug Addiction in 178 Patients: Preliminary Results," *Child Abuse & Neglect* 6, no. 4 (1982): 383–87, DOI:10.1016/0145-2134(82)90081-3.

31. Kristen W. Springer, Jennifer Sheridan, Daphne Kuo, and Molly Carnes, "The Long-term Health Outcomes of Childhood Abuse," *Journal of*

General Internal Medicine 18, no. 10 (2003): 864–70, DOI:10.1046/j.1525-1497.2003.20918.x.

32. Alec Roy, "Childhood Trauma and Neuroticism as an Adult: Possible Implication for the Development of the Common Psychiatric Disorders and Suicidal Behaviour," *Psychological Medicine* 32, no. 8 (2002): 1471–74, DOI:10.1017/S0033291702006566.

APPENDIX B

1. David K. Smith, Bruce D. Hale, and David J. Collins, "Measurement of Exercise Dependence in Bodybuilders," *Journal of Sport Medicine and Physical Fitness* 38, no. 1 (1998): 66–74.

2. Kata Mónok, Krisztina Berczik, Róbert Urbán, Attila Szabó, Mark D. Griffiths, Judit Farkas, Anna Magi, Andrea Eisinger, Tamás Kurimay, Gyöngyi Kökönyei, Bernadette Kun, Borbála Paksi, and Zsolt Demetrovics, "Psychometric Properties and Concurrent Validity of Two Exercise Addiction Measures: A Population Wide Study," *Psychology of Sport & Exercise* 13, no. 6 (2012): 739–46, DOI:10.1016/j.psychsport.2012.06.003.

3. Annabel Terry, Attila Szabó, and Mark D. Griffiths, "The Exercise Addiction Inventory: A New Brief Screening Tool," *Addiction Research and Theory* 12, no. 5 (2004): 489–99, DOI:10.1080/16066350310001637363.

4. Mark D. Griffiths, "Nicotine, Tobacco and Addiction," *Nature* 384, no. 6604 (1996): 18.

5. Annabel Terry, Attila Szabó, and Mark D. Griffiths, "The Exercise Addiction Inventory: A New Brief Screening Tool," *Addiction Research and Theory* 12, no. 5 (2004): 489–99, DOI:10.1080/16066350310001637363.

6. Heather Hausenblas and Danielle Symons Downs, "How Much Is Too Much? The Development and Validation of the Exercise Dependence Scale," *Psychology & Health* 17, no. 4 (2001): 387–404, DOI:10.1080/0887044022000004894.

7. Danielle Symons Downs, Heather A. Hausenblas, and Claudio R. Nigg, "Factorial Validity and Psychometric Examination of the Exercise Dependence Scale—Revised," *Measurement in Physical Education and Exercise Science* 8, no. 4 (2004): 183–201, DOI:10.1207/s15327841mpee0804_1.

8. Lorin Taranis, Stephen Touyz, and Caroline Meyer, "Disordered Eating and Exercise: Development and Preliminary Validation of the Compulsive Exercise Test (CET)," *European Eating Disorders Review* 19, no. 3 (2011): 256–68, DOI:10.1002/erv.1108.

9. Lorin Taranis, Stephen Touyz, and Caroline Meyer, "Disordered Eating and Exercise: Development and Preliminary Validation of the Compulsive Ex-

ercise Test (CET)," *European Eating Disorders Review* 19, no. 3 (2011): 256–68, DOI:10.1002/erv.1108.

BIBLIOGRAPHY

Aarenstein, Anna. "Home Fitness Reaches Mind-boggling Sales Explosion." *Gainesville Sun*, June 24, 1984.

A.D.A.M. Medical Encyclopedia. "Metabolic Acidosis." PubMed Health. www.ncbi.nlm.nih.gov/pubmedhealth/PMH0001376. Last modified November 17, 2011.

Adlercreutz, Herman, Mikko Härkönen, Kimmo Kuoppasalmi, Hannu Näveri, Ilpo Huhtaniemi, Heiki O. Tikkanen, Kari Remes, Adriano Dessypris, and Jukka Karvonen. "Effect of Training on Plasma Anabolic and Catabolic Steroid Hormones and Their Response during Physical Exercise." *International Journal of Sports Medicine* 7, suppl. no. 1 (1986): 27–28. DOI:10.1055/s-2008-1025798.

Aidman, Eugene V., and Simon Woollard. "The Influence of Self-reported Exercise Addiction on Acute Emotional and Physiological Responses to Brief Exercise Deprivation." *Psychology of Sport and Exercise* 4, no. 3 (2003): 225–36. DOI:10.1016/S1469-0292(02)00003-1.

Allport, Floyd Henry. "The J-curve Hypothesis of Conforming Behavior." *Journal of Social Psychology* 5 (1934): 141–83.

American Association of Neurological Surgeons. "Sports-related Head Injury." www.aans.org/Patient Information/Conditions and Treatments/Sports-Related Injury.aspx. Last modified December 2011. Accessed March 26, 2014.

American College of Sports Medicine. "Research Yields Fitness Motivation Tips for a Healthy New Year." www.acsm.org/about-acsm/media-room/news-releases/2011/08/01/research-yields-fitness-motivation-tips-for-a-healthy-new-year. Last modified August 1, 2011. Accessed March 25, 2014.

———. "The Female Athlete Triad." www.acsm.org/docs/brochures/the-female-athlete-triad.pdf. Last modified 2011.

American Orthopaedic Society for Sports Medicine. "Overuse Injuries." www.sportsmed.org/uploadedFiles/Content/Patient/Sports_Tips/ST%20Overuse%20Injuries%2008.pdf. Last modified 2008.

American Psychiatric Association. *Diagnostic and Statistical Manual of Mental Disorders.* Washington, DC: American Psychiatric Association, 2013.

American Society of Addiction Medicine, "Public Policy Statement: Definition of Addiction." www.asam.org/for-the-public/definition-of-addiction. Last modified April 19, 2011. Accessed February 22, 2014.

Anonymous. "The Cult of the Gym: The New Puritans." *The Economist*. December 19, 2002. www.economist.com/node/1487649. Accessed February 24, 2014.

———. "Athletics in Schools." *The Popular Science Monthly*. Volume 16 (March 1880): 677–84.

Arbour, Kelly P., and Kathleen A. Martin Ginnis. "Effects of Exposure of Muscular and Hypermuscular Images on Young Men's Muscularity Dissatisfaction and Body Dissatisfaction." *Body Image* 3, no. 2 (2006): 153–62. DOI:10.1016/j.bodyim.2006.03.004.

Ashton, Jennifer. "Addicted to Exercise." Health and Wellness. CBS News. November 2, 2009. www.cbsnews.com/videos/addicted-to-exercise. Accessed April 2, 2014.

Baekeland, Frederick. "Exercise Deprivation: Sleep and Psychological Reactions." *Archives of General Psychiatry* 22, no. 4 (1970): 365–69. DOI:10.1001/archpsyc.1970.01740 280077014.

Baler, Ruben D., and Nora D. Volkow. "Drug Addiction: The Neurobiology of Disrupted Self-control." *Trends in Molecular Medicine* 12, no. 12 (2006): 559–66. DOI:10.1016/j.molmed.2006.10.005.

Bamber, Diane J., Ian M. Cockerill, S. Rodgers, and Doug Carroll. "Diagnostic Criteria for Exercise Dependence in Women." *British Journal of Sports Medicine* 37, no. 5 (2003): 393–400. DOI:10.1136/bjsm.37.5.393.

Barnes, George E., Robert P. Murray, David Patton, Peter M. Bentler, and Robert E. Anderson. *The Addiction-prone Personality*. New York: Kluwer Academic/Plenum Publishers, 2000.

Baum, Andrew, and Donna M. Polsusnzy. "Health Psychology: Mapping Biobehavioral Contributions to Health and Illness." *Annual Review of Psychology* 50 (1999): 137–63. DOI:10.1146/annurev.psych.50.1.137.

Baum, Sandy, Jennifer Ma, and Kathleen Payea. "Health Benefits: Exercise." *Education Pays 2013: The Benefits of Higher Education for Individuals and Society*. New York: The College Board, 2013.

Baylor, L. S., and Anthony C. Hackney. "Resting Thyroid and Leptin Hormone Changes in Women Following Intense, Prolonged Exercise Training." *European Journal of Applied Physiology* 88, nos. 4–5 (2003): 480–84.

Beh, Helen C., Sarah Mathers, and John Holden. "EEG Correlates of Exercise Dependency." *International Journal of Psychophysiology* 23, nos. 1–2 (1996): 121–28. DOI:10.1016/0167-8760(96)00039-6.

Berczik, Krisztina, Attila Szabó, Mark D. Griffiths, Tamás Kurimay, Bernadette Kun, Róbert Urbán, and Zsolt Demetrovics. "Exercise Addiction: Symptoms, Diagnosis, Epidemiology, and Etiology." *Substance Use & Misuse* 47, no. 4 (2012): 403–17. DOI:10.3109/10826084.2011.639120.

Birditt, Kira S., Karen L. Fingerman, and David M. Almeida. "Age Differences in Exposure and Reactions to Interpersonal Tensions: A Daily Diary Study." *Psychology and Aging* 20, no. 2 (2005): 330–40. DOI:10.1037/0882-7974.20.2.330.

Bishop, Phillip A., Eric Jones, and Krista A. Woods. "Recovery from Training: A Brief Review." *Journal of Strength & Conditioning Research* 22, no. 3 (2008): 1015–24. DOI:10.1519/JSC.0b013e31816eb518.

Blaydon, Michelle J., and Koenraad J. Lindner. "Eating Disorders and Exercise Dependence in Triathletes." *Eating Disorders* 10, no. 1 (2002): 49–60, DOI:10.1080/106402602753573559.

Bolding, Graham, Lorraine Sherr, and Jonathan Elford. "Use of Anabolic Steroids and Associated Health Risks among Gay Men Attending London Gyms." *Addiction* 97, no. 2 (2002): 195–203. DOI:10.1046/j.1360-0442.2002.00031.xs.

Bostwick, J. Michael. "Internet Sex Addiction Treated with Naltrexone." *Mayo Clinic Proceedings* 83, no. 2 (2008): 226–30.

Bourdieu, Pierre. *Distinction: A Social Critique of the Judgment of Taste*. Cambridge, MA: Harvard University Press, 1984.

Bovens, Astrid, Geert Janssen, H. G. W. Vermeer, Jean H. Hoeberigs, Marie P. Janssen, and Frans T. J. Verstappen. "Occurrence of Running Injuries in Adults Following a Supervised Training Program." *International Journal of Sports Medicine* 10, no. S3 (1989): S186–S190. DOI:10.1055/s-2007-1024970.

Boyden, Thomas W., Richard W. Pamenter, Thomas C. Rotkis, Philip Stanforth, and Jack H. Wilmore. "Thyroidal Changes Associated with Endurance Training in Women." *Medicine & Science in Sports & Exercise* 16, no. 3 (1984): 234–46.

Brooks, Douglas. *The Complete Book of Personal Training.* Champaign, IL: Human Kinetics, 2004.

Brownell, Kelly D. "Dieting and the Search for the Perfect Body: Where Physiology and Culture Collide." *Behavior Therapy* 22, no. 1 (1991): 1–12. DOI:10.1016/S0005-7894(05)80239-4.

Buckley, William E., Charles E. Yesalis III, Karl E. Friedl, William A. Anderson, Andrea L. Streit, and James E. Wright. "Estimated Prevalence of Anabolic Steroid Use among Male High School Seniors." *The Journal of the American Medical Association* 260, no. 23 (1988): 3441–45. DOI:10.1001/jama.1988.03410230059028.

Buckworth, Janet, Rod K. Dishman, Patrick J. O'Connor, and Phillip D. Tomporowski. *Exercise Psychology.* 2nd ed. Champaign, IL: Human Kinetics, 2013.

Bulik, Cynthia M., and Nancy D. Berkman. "Eating Disorders: Newer Practice Guidelines Reinforce Severity of Conditions but Still Reflect Deficits in Knowledge Base." National Guideline Clearinghouse. February 25, 2008. www.guideline.gov/expert/printView.aspx?id=16450. Accessed: March 17, 2014.

Burton, Deborah A., Keith Stokes, and George M. Hall. "Physiological Effects of Exercise." *Continuing Education in Anaesthesia, Critical Care & Pain* 4, no. 6 (2004): 185–88. DOI:10.1093/bjaceaccp/mkh050.

Caldwell, Nolan, Tanja Srebotnjak, Tiffany Wang, and Renee Hsia. "'How Much Will I Get Charged for This?' Patient Charges for Top Ten Diagnoses in the Emergency Department." *PLOSone* 8, no. 1 (2013): e55491. DOI:10.1371/journal.pone.0055491.

Carnes, Patrick J., Robert E. Murray, and Louis Charpentier. "Bargains with Chaos: Sex Addicts and Addiction Interaction Disorder." *Sexual Addiction and Compulsivity: The Journal of Treatment and Prevention* 12, nos. 2–3 (2005): 79–120. DOI:10.1080/10720160500201371.

Carrier, Claire. "Addiction to Muscular Exercise: The Limit of Somatopsychology When Linked to Sport." *Addictions et travail* VST, no. 98 (2008): 35–41.

Cattarin, Jill A., Kevin Thompson, Carmen Thomas, and Robyn Williams. "Body Image, Mood, and Televised Images of Attractiveness: The Role of Social Comparison." *Journal of Social and Clinical Psychology* 19, no. 2 (2000): 220–39. DOI:10.1521/jscp.2000.19.2.220.

Centers for Disease Control and Prevention. "Healthy Weight—It's Not a Diet, It's a Lifestyle!" www.cdc.gov/healthyweight/assessing/bmi/adult_bmi. Last modified September 13, 2011. Accessed February 22, 2014.

———. "How Much Physical Activity Do You Need?" www.cdc.gov/physicalactivity/everyone/guidelines/index.html. Last modified March 30, 2011. Accessed April 23, 2014.

———. "National Hospital Ambulatory Medical Care Survey: 2010 Emergency Department Summary Tables." www.cdc.gov/nchs/data/ahcd/nhamcs_emergency/2010_ed_web_tables.pdf. Accessed March 26, 2014.

———. "Participation in Leisure-time Aerobic and Muscle-strengthening Activities That Meet the Federal 2008 Physical Activity Guidelines for Americans among Adults Aged 18 and Over, by Selected Characteristics: United States, Selected Years 1998–2012." www.cdc.gov/nchs/data/hus/2012/067.pdf. Accessed March 28, 2014.

Chadwick, Paul, Stephanie Hughes, Daphne Russell, Ian Russel, and Dave Dagnan. "Mindfulness Groups for Distressing Voices and Paranoia: A Replication and Randomized Feasibility Trial." *Behavioural and Cognitive Psychotherapy* 37, no. 4 (2009): 403–12. DOI:10.1017/S1352465809990166.

Christesen, Paul, and Donald G. Kyle. *A Companion to Sport and Spectacle in Greek and Roman Antiquity.* Malden, MA: Wiley-Blackwell, 2014.

Clarkson, Priscilla M. "Exertional Rhabdomyolysis and Acute Renal Failure in Marathon Runners." *Sports Medicine* 37 nos. 4–5 (2007): 361–63. DOI:10.2165/00007256-200737040-00022.

Clays, Els, Dirk De Bacquer, Heidi Janssens, Bart De Clercq, Annalisa Casini, Lutgart Braeckman, France Kittel, Guy De Backer, and Andreas Holtermann. "The Association between Leisure Time Physical Activity and Coronary Heart Disease among Men with

Different Work Demands: A Prospective Cohort Study." *European Journal of Epidemiology* 28, no. 3 (2013): 241–47. DOI:10.1007/s10654-013-9764-4.

Cockell, Sarah J., Josie Geller, and Wolfgang Linden. "Decisional Balance in Anorexia Nervosa: Capitalizing on Ambivalence." *European Eating Disorders Review* 11, no. 2 (2003): 75–89.

Cohen, Frederick S., and Judianne Densen-Gerber. "A Study of the Relationship between Child Abuse and Drug Addiction in 178 Patients: Preliminary Results." *Child Abuse & Neglect* 6, no. 4 (1982): 383–87. DOI:10.1016/0145-2134(82)90081-3.

Conn, Judith M., Joseph L. Annest, and Julie Gilchrist. "Sports and Recreation Related Injury Episodes in the U.S. Population, 1997–99." *Injury Prevention* 9, no. 2 (2003): 117–23. DOI:10.1136/ip.9.2.117.

Cook, Brian, Heather Hausenblas, Daniel Tuccitto, and Peter R. Giacobbi. "Eating Disorders and Exercise: A Structural Equation Modeling Analysis of a Conceptual Model." *European Eating Disorders Review* 19, no. 3. (2011): 216–25. DOI:10.1002/erv.1111.

Cook, Brian, Trisha M. Karr, Christie Zunker, James E. Mitchell, Ron Thompson, Roberta Sherman, Ross D. Crosby, Li Cao, Ann Erickson, and Stephen A. Wonderlich. "Primary and Secondary Exercise Dependence in a Community-based Sample of Road Race Runners." *Journal of Sport & Exercise Psychology* 35, no. 5 (2013): 464–69.

Costa, Paul T., and Robert R. McCrae. *Revised NEO Personality Inventory (NEO-PI-R) and NEO Five-factor Inventory (NEO-FFI) Professional Manual.* Odessa, FL: Psychological Assessment Resources, 1992.

Costa, Sebastiano, Heather A. Hausenblas, Patrizia Oliva, Francesca Cuzzocrea, and Rosalba Larcan. "The Role of Age, Gender, Mood States and Exercise Frequency on Exercise Dependence." *Journal of Behavioral Addictions* 2, no. 4 (2013): 216–23. DOI:10.1556/JBA.2.2013.014.

Costa, Sebastiano, and Patrizia Oliva. "Examining Relationship between Personality Characteristics and Exercise Dependence." *Review of Psychology* 19, no. 1 (2012): 5–12.

Crocker, Jennifer. "The Costs of Seeking Self-esteem." *Journal of Social Issues* 58, no. 3 (2002): 597–615.

Crowther, Nigel B. *Sport in Ancient Times.* Westport, CT: Praeger Publications, 2007.

Cully, Jeffrey A., and Andra L. Teten. *A Therapist's Guide to Brief Cognitive Behavioral Therapy.* Houston, TX: Department of Veterans Affairs South Central MIRECC, 2008.

Dahl, Melissa. "Gym-goers Trip, Flip, and Fall in Pursuit of Fitness." NBCNews.com. www.nbcnews.com/id/35127528/ns/health-fitness/t/gym-goers-trip-flip-fall-pursuit-fitness. Last modified January 1, 2010. Accessed March 26, 2014.

Davis, Caroline, and Michael Cowles. "Body Image and Exercise: A Study of Relationships and Comparisons between Physically Active Men and Women." *Sex Roles* 25, nos. 1–2 (1991): 33–44. DOI:10.1007/BF00289315.

Deci, Edward L., and Richard M. Ryan. "Human Autonomy: The Basis for True Self-esteem." In *Efficacy, agency, and self-esteem,* edited by Michael H. Kernis, 31–49. New York: Plenum, 1995.

De Coverley Veale, David. "Exercise Dependence." *British Journal of Addiction* 82, no. 7 (1987): 735–40. DOI:10.1111/j.1360-0443.1987.tb01539.x.

Dietrich, Arne, and William F. McDaniel. "Endocannabinoids and Exercise." *British Journal of Sports Medicine* 38, no. 5 (2004): 536–41. DOI:10.1136/bjsm.2004.011718.

Di Nicola, Marco, Giovanni Martinotti, Marianna Mazza, Daniela Tedeschi, Gino Pozzi, and Luigi Janiri. "Quetiapine as Add-on Treatment for Bipolar I Disorder with Comorbid Compulsive Buying and Physical Exercise Addiction." *Progress in Neuro-psychopharmacology & Biological Psychiatry* 34, no. 4 (2010): 713–14. DOI:10.1016/j.pnpbp.2010.03.013.

Emler, Nicholas. *Self-esteem: The Costs and Causes of Low Self-worth.* York, UK: Joseph Rowntree Foundation, 2001.

Erickson, Kirk I., Michelle W. Vossb, Ruchika Shaurya Prakash, Chandramallika Basak, Attila Szabó, Laura Chaddock, Jennifer S. Kim, Susie Heo, Heloisa Alves, Siobhan M. White, Thomas R. Wojcicki, Emily Mailey, Victoria J. Vieira, Stephen A. Martin, Brandt D. Pence, Jeffrey A. Woods, Edward McAuley, and Arthur F. Kramer. "Exercise Training

Increases Size of Hippocampus and Improves Memory." *Proceedings of the National Academy of Sciences* 108, no. 7 (2011): 3017–22. DOI:10.1073/pnas.1015950108.

Fairburn, Christopher, Zafra Cooper, and Roz Shafran. "Cognitive Behaviour Therapy for Eating Disorders: A 'Transdiagnostic' Theory and Treatment." *Behaviour Research and Therapy* 41, no. 5 (2003): 509–28. DOI:10.1016/S0005-7967(02)00088-8.

Fitspoholic. Daily Motivation. http://fitspoholic.tumblr.com/tagged/fitspoholic. Accessed March 25, 2014.

Freeman, Kenneth John. *Schools of Hellas: An Essay on the Practice and Theory of Ancient Greek Education from 600 to 300 B.C.* London: St. Martin's Press, 1907.

Freeman, William H. *Physical Education, Exercise and Sport Science in a Changing Society.* 7th ed. Burlington, MA: Jones & Bartlett Learning, 2012.

Freimuth, Marilyn, Sandy Moniz, and Shari R. Kim. "Clarifying Exercise Addiction: Differential Diagnosis, Co-occurring Disorders, and Phases of Addiction." *International Journal of Environmental Research and Public Health* 8, no. 10 (2011): 4069–81. DOI:10.3390/ijerph8104069.

Frost, Randy O., and Gail Steketee. "Perfectionism in Obsessive-compulsive Disorder Patients." *Behaviour Research and Therapy* 35, no. 4 (1997): 291–96. DOI:10.1016/S0005-7967(96)00108-8.

Furnham, Adrian, Nicola Badmin, and Ian Sneade. "Body Image Dissatisfaction: Gender Differences in Eating Attitudes, Self-esteem, and Reasons for Exercise." *The Journal of Psychology* 13, no. 6 (2002): 581–96.

Gale Group. "Physical Fitness Facilities SIC 7991 Industry Reports." *Highbeam Business Report.* http://business.highbeam.com/industry-reports/personal/physical-fitness-facilities. Last modified 2014. Accessed February 24, 2014.

George, Alan J. "Central Nervous System Stimulants." *Best Practice & Research Clinical Endocrinology & Metabolism* 14, no. 1 (2000): 79–88. DOI:10.1053/beem.2000.0055.

Gilchrist, Julie, Karen E. Thomas, Likang Xu, Lisa C. McGuire, and Victor Coronado. "Nonfatal Sports and Recreation Related Traumatic Brain Injuries among Children and Adolescents Treated in Emergency Departments in the United States, 2001–2009." *Morbidity and Mortality Weekly Report* 60, no. 39 (2011): 1337–42.

Glasser, William. *Positive Addictions.* New York: Harper Colophon, 1976.

Goldfarb, Allan H., and Athanasios Z. Jamurtas. "Beta-endorphin Response to Exercise: An Update." *Sports Medicine* 24, no. 1 (1997): 8–16. DOI:10.2165/00007256-199724010-00002.

Goldfarb, Lori A., Elisabeth M. Dykens, and Meg Gerrard. "The Goldfarb Fear of Fat Scale." *Journal of Personality Assessment* 49, no. 3 (1985): 329–32. DOI:10.1207/s15327752jpa4903_21.

Goodman, Aviel. "Neurobiology of Addiction: An Integrative Review." *Biochemical Pharmacology* 75, no. 1 (2008): 266–322. DOI:10.1016/j.bcp.2007.07.030.

Goodman, Linnea R., and Michelle P. Warren. "The Female Athlete and Menstrual Function." *Current Opinion in Obstetrics and Gynecology* 17, no. 15 (2005): 446–70.

Gorla, Kiranmai, and Maju Mathews. "Pharmacological Treatment of Eating Disorders," *Psychiatry* 2, no. 6 (2005): 42–48.

Grieve, Frederick G., Natalie Truba, and Sandy Bowersox. "Etiology, Assessment, and Treatment of Muscle Dysmorphia." *Journal of Cognitive Psychotherapy* 23, no. 4 (2009): 306–14.

Griffiths, Mark D. "Nicotine, Tobacco and Addiction." *Nature* 384, no. 6604 (1996): 18.

Griffiths, Mark D. Attila Szabó, and Annabel Terry. "The Exercise Addiction Inventory: A Quick and Easy Screening Tool for Health Practitioners." *British Journal of Sports Medicine* 39, no. 6 (2005): 30–31.

Grogan, Sarah, and Nicola Wainwright. "Growing Up in the Culture of Slenderness: Girls' Experiences of Body Dissatisfaction." *Women's Studies International Forum* 19, no. 6 (1996): 665–73. DOI:10.1016/S0277-5395(96)00076-3.

Gull, William. "Anorexia Nervosa (Apepsia Hysteria)." *Transactions of the Clinical Society of London* 7 (1874): 22–28.

Hamer, Mark, and Costas I. Karageorghis. "Psychobiological Mechanisms of Exercise Dependence." *Sports Medicine* 37, no. 6 (2007): 477–84. DOI:10.2165/00007256-200737060-00002.

Hamilton, Kelly, and Gören Waller. "Media Influences on Body Size Estimation in Anorexia and Bulimia: An Experimental Study." *The British Journal of Psychiatry* 162 (1993): 837–40.

Hansen, Cheryl J., Larry C. Stevens, and Richard J. Coast. "Exercise Duration and Mood State: How Much Is Enough to Feel Better?" *Health Psychology* 20, no. 4 (2001): 267–75. DOI:10.1037/0278-6133.20.4.267.

Harvard Health Publications. "The Addicted Brain." *Harvard Mental Health Letter*. July 2004. www.health.harvard.edu/newsweek/The_addicted_brain.htm. Accessed February 22, 2014.

Hausenblas, Heather A., Brian J. Cook, and Nickles I. Chittester. "Can Exercise Treat Eating Disorders?" *Exercise and Sport Sciences Reviews* 36, no. 1 (2008): 43–47.

Hausenblas, Heather A., Britton W. Brewer, and Judy L. Van Raalte. "Self-presentation and Exercise." *Journal of Applied Sport Psychology* 16, no. 1 (2004): 3–18. DOI:10.1080/10413200490260026.

Hausenblas, Heather A., and Danielle Symons Downs. "Exercise Dependence: A Systematic Review." *Psychology of Sport and Exercise* 3, no. 2 (2002): 89–123. DOI:10.1016/S1469-0292(00)00015-7.

———. "Relationship among Sex, Imagery and Exercise Dependence Symptoms." *Psychology of Addictive Behaviors* 16, no. 2 (2002): 169–72. DOI:10.1037/0893-164X.16.2.169.

———. "How Much Is Too Much? The Development and Validation of the Exercise Dependence Scale." *Psychology & Health* 17, no. 4 (2001): 387–404. DOI:10.1080/0887044022000004894.

Hausenblas, Heather A., Debbie Saha, Pamela Jean Dubyak, and Stephen Douglas Anton. "Saffron (*Crocus Sativus L.*) and Major Depressive Disorder: A Meta-analysis of Randomized Clinical Trials." *Journal of Integrative Medicine* 11, no. 6 (2013): 377–83. DOI:10.3736/jintegrmed2013056.

Hausenblas, Heather A., and Elizabeth A. Fallon. "Exercise and Body Image: A Meta-analysis." *Psychology & Health* 21, no. 1 (2006): 33–47. DOI:10.1080/14768320500105270.

———. "Relationship among Body Image, Exercise Behavior, and Exercise Dependence Symptoms." *International Journal of Eating Disorders* 32, no. 2 (2002): 179–85. DOI:10.1002/eat.10071.

Hausenblas, Heather A., and Peter Giacobbi. "Relationship between Exercise Dependence Symptoms and Personality." *Personality and Individual Differences* 36, no. 6 (2004): 1265–73. DOI:10.1016/S0191-8869(03)00214-9.

Haylett, Samantha A., Geoffrey M. Stephenson, and Robert M. H. LeFever. "Covariation of Addictive Behaviors: A Study of Addictive Orientation Using the Shorter PROMIS Questionnaire." *Addictive Behaviors* 29, no. 1 (2004): 61–71. DOI:10.1016/S0306-4603(03)00083-2.

Hayward, Peter. *Intermediate GNVQ Leisure and Tourism Student Book without Options*. Oxford: Heinemann Educational Publishers, 2000.

Hepworth, Julie. *The Social Construction of Anorexia Nervosa*. London: Sage, 1999.

Hillman, Charles H., Kirk I. Erickson, and Arthur F. Kramer. "Be Smart, Exercise Your Heart: Exercise Effects on Brain and Cognition." *Nature Reviews Neuroscience* 9, no. 1 (2008): 58–65. DOI:10.1038/nrn2298.

Hind, Karen. "Recovery of Bone Mineral Density and Fertility in a Former Amenorrheic Athlete." *Journal of Sports Science & Medicine* 7, no. 3 (2008): 415–18.

Hooper, Sue L., Laurel Traeger Mackinnon, Richard D. Gordon, and Anthony W. Bachmann. "Hormonal Responses of Elite Swimmers to Overtraining." *Medicine and Science in Sports and Exercise* 25, no. 6 (1993): 741–47.

Hootman, Jennifer M., Carol A. Macera, Barbara E. Ainsworth, Malissa Martin, Cheryl L. Addy, and Steven N. Blair. "Association among Physical Activity Level, Cardiorespiratory

Fitness, and Risk of Musculoskeletal Injury." *American Journal of Epidemiology* 154, no. 3 (2001): 251–58. DOI:10.1093/aje/154.3.251.

International Health, Racquet, and Sportsclub Association. "58.5 Million Americans Utilize Health Clubs." www.ihrsa.org/media-center/2013/5/8/585-million-americans-utilize-health-clubs.html. Accessed February 24, 2014.

———. "Consumer Research." www.ihrsa.org/consumer-research. Accessed February 24, 2014.

———. *The Global Report, 2013.*

Jacobs, Durand F. "A General Theory of Addictions: A New Theoretical Model." *Journal of Gambling Behavior* 2, no. 1 (1986): 15–31.

Janal, Malvin, Edward W. D. Colt, W. Crawford Clark, and Murray Glusman. "Pain Sensitivity, Mood and Plasma Endocrine Levels Following Long-distance Running: Effects of Naloxone." *Pain* 19, no. 1 (1984): 13–25. DOI:10.1016/0304-3959(84)90061-7.

Janet, Pierre. *The Major Symptoms of Hysteria: Fifteen Lectures Given in the Medical School of Harvard University.* London: Macmillan, 1920.

Janowsky, David S., Liyi Hong, Shirley Morter, and Laura Howe. "Underlying Personality Differences between Alcohol/Substance-use Disorder Patients with and without an Affective Disorder." *Alcohol & Alcoholism* 34, no. 3 (1999): 370–77. DOI:10.1093/alcalc/34.3.370.

Johnson, Mary B., and Steven M. Thiese. "A Review of Overtraining Syndrome—Recognizing the Signs and Symptoms." *Journal of Athletic Training* 27, no. 4 (1992): 352–54.

Jones, Emmett. "Athletic Apparel Revenue to Reach $180 Billion a Year by 2018." *Sports Business Digest.* http://sportsbusinessdigest.com/2013/03/athletic-apparel-revenue-to-reach-180-billion-a-year-by-2018. Last modified March 5, 2013. Accessed March 26, 2014.

Juarascio, Adrienne S., Evan M. Forman, and James D. Herbert. "Acceptance and Commitment Therapy versus Cognitive Therapy for the Treatment of Comorbid Eating Pathology." *Behavior Modification* 34, no. 2 (2010): 175–90.

Kamen, Gary. *Foundations of Exercise Science.* Philadelphia: Lippincott Williams & Wilkins, 2001.

Karim, Reef, and Priya Chaudhri. "Behavioral Addictions: An Overview." *Journal of Psychoactive Drugs* 44, no. 1 (2012): 5–17. DOI:10.1080/02791072.2012.662859.

Kern, Laurence. "Relation entre la dépendance à l'exercice physique et les cinq dimensions de la personnalité." *L'Encéphale* 36, no. 3 (2010): 212–18. DOI:10.1016/j.encep.2009.06.007.

Kerr, Zachary Y., Christy L. Collins, and R. Dawn Comstock. "Epidemiology of Weight Training–related Injuries Presenting to United States Emergency Departments." *The American Journal of Medicine* 38, no. 4 (2010): 765–61. DOI:10.1177/0363546509351560.

Kilpatrick, Dean G., Deborah A. McAlhany, R. Layton McCurdy, Darlene Shaw, and John C. Roitzsch. "Aging, Alcoholism, Anxiety, and Sensation Seeking: An Exploratory Investigation." *Addictive Behavior* 7, no. 1 (1982): 97–100. DOI:10.1016/0306-4603(82)90033-8.

Kim, Jonathan H., Rajeev Malhotra, George Chiampas, Pierre d'Hemecourt, Chris Troyanos, John Cianca, Rex N. Smith, Thomas J. Wang, William O. Roberts, Paul D. Thompson, and Aaron L. Baggish. "Cardiac Arrest during Long-distance Running Races." *The New England Journal of Medicine* 366, no. 2 (2012): 130–40. DOI:10.1056/NEJMoa1106468.

Kirk, David, Doune Macdonald, and Mary O'Sullivan. *Handbook of Physical Education.* London: Sage, 2006.

Kirkwood, Graham, Hagen Rampes, Veronica Tuffrey, Janet Richardson, and Karen Pilkington. "Yoga for Anxiety: A Systematic Review of the Research Evidence." *British Journal of Sports Medicine* 39, no. 12 (2005): 884–91. DOI:10.1136/bjsm.2005.018069.

Klein, Diane A., Andrew S. Bennett, Janet Schebendach, Richard W. Foltin, Michael J. Devlin, and B. Timothy Walsh. "Exercise 'Addiction' in Anorexia Nervosa: Model Development and Pilot Data." *CNS Spectrums* 9, no. 7 (2004): 531–37.

Kristeller, Jean L., Ruth A. Baer, and Ruth Quillian-Wolever. "Mindfulness-based Approaches to Eating Disorders." In *Mindfulness-based Treatment Approaches: Clinician's*

Guide to Evidence Base and Applications, edited by Ruth A. Baer, 75–91. London: Elsevier, 2006.

Langlois, Jean A., Wesley Rutland-Brown, and Marlena M. Wald. "The Epidemiology and Impact of Traumatic Brain Injury: A Brief Overview." *Journal of Head Trauma Rehabilitation* 21, no. 5 (2006): 375–78.

Lecomte, Dominique, Paul Fornes, Pierre Fouret, and Guy Nicolas. "Isolated Myocardial Fibrosis as a Cause of Sudden Cardiac Death and Its Possible Relation to Myocarditis." *Journal of Forensic Sciences* 38, no. 3 (1993): 617–21.

Lee, Duck-chul, Russell R. Pate, Carl J. Lavie, and Steven N. Blair. "Running and All-cause Mortality Risk: Is More Better?" ACSM Annual Meeting: World Congress on Exercise in Medicine, May 29–June 2, 2012, San Francisco, CA: 3471.

Lejoyeux, Michel, Marine Avril, Charlotte Richoux, Houcine Embouazza, and Fabrizia Nivoli. "Prevalence of Exercise Dependence and Other Behavioral Addictions among Clients of a Parisian Fitness Room." *Comprehensive Psychiatry* 49, no. 4 (2008): 353–58. DOI:10.1016/j.comppsych.2007.12.005.

Lerner, Richard M., Stuart A. Karabenick, and Joyce L. Stuart. "Relations among Physical Attractiveness, Body Attitudes, and Self-concept in Male and Female College Students." *The Journal of Psychology: Interdisciplinary and Applied* 85, no. 1 (1973): 119–29. DOI:10.1080/00223980.1973.9923870.

Lichtenstein, Mia Beck, Erik Christiansen, Ask Elklit, Niels Bilenberg, and René Klinky Støving. "Exercise Addiction: A Study of Eating Disorder Symptoms, Quality of Life, Personality Traits and Attachment Styles." *Psychiatry Research* 215, no. 2 (2014): 410–16. DOI:10.1016/j.psychres.2013.11.010.

Lindwall, Magnus, and Kathleen A. Martin Ginis. "Moving towards a Favorable Image: The Self-presentational Benefits of Exercise and Physical Activity." *Scandinavian Journal of Psychology* 47, no. 3 (2006): 209–17.

Line, Robin L., and George S. Rust. "Acute Exertional Rhabdomyolysis." *Family Physician* 52, no. 2 (1995): 502–6.

Long, Clive G., Jenny Smith, Marie Midgley, and Tony Cassidy. "Over-exercising in Anorexic and Normal Samples: Behaviour and Attitudes." *Journal of Mental Health* 2, no. 4 (1993): 321–27. DOI:10.3109/09638239309016967.

Loucks, Anne. "Refutation of 'the Myth of the Female Athlete Triad.'" *British Journal of Sports Medicine* 41, no. 1 (2007): 55–57.

MacAndrew, Craig. "Male Alcoholics, Secondary Psychopathy and Eysenck's Theory of Personality." *Personality and Individual Differences* 1, no. 2 (1980): 151–60. DOI:10.1016/0191-8869(80)90033-1.

MacLaren, Vance V., and Lisa A. Best. "Multiple Addictive Behaviors in Young Adults: Student Norms for the Shorter PROMIS Questionnaire." *Addictive Behaviors* 35, no. 3 (2010): 252–55. DOI:10.1016/j.addbeh.2009.09.023.

Magai, Carol, Nathan S. Consedine, Yulia S. Krivoshekova, Elizabeth Kudadje-Gyamfi, and Renee McPherson. "Emotion Experience and Expression across the Adult Life Span: Insights from a Multimodal Assessment Study." *Psychology and Aging* 21, no. 2 (2006): 303–17. DOI:10.1037/0882-7974.21.2.303.

Maguire, Jennifer Smith. "Body Lessons: Fitness Publishing and the Cultural Production of the Fitness Consumer." *International Review for the Sociology of Sport* 37, nos. 3–4 (2002): 449–64. DOI:10.1177/1012690020037004896.

Maron, Barry J. "Hypertrophic Cardiomyopathy: A Systematic Review." *The Journal of the American Medical Association: Clinical Cardiology* 287, no. 10 (2002): 1308–20. DOI:10.1001/jama.287.10.1308.

Maron, Barry J., and Antonio Pelliccia. "The Heart of Trained Athletes: Cardiac Remodeling and the Risk of Sports, Including Sudden Death." *Circulation* 114, no. 15 (2006): 1633–44. DOI:10.1161/CIRCULATIONAHA.106.613562.

Martin, Eric D., and Kenneth J. Sher. "Family History of Alcoholism, Alcohol Use Disorders and the Five-factor Model of Personality." *Journal of Studies on Alcohol* 55, no. 1 (1994): 81–90.

McCabe, Marita P., and Lina A. Ricciardelli. "Body Image Dissatisfaction among Males across the Lifespan: A Review of Past Literature." *Journal of Psychosomatic Research* 56, no. 6 (2004): 675–85. DOI:10.1016/S0022-3999(03)00129-6.

McClelland, John. *Body and Mind: Sport in Europe from the Roman Empire to the Renaissance*. New York: Routledge, 2007.

McCullough, Peter A., Kavitha M. Chinnaiyan, Michael J. Gallagher, James M. Colar, Timothy Geddes, Jeffrey M. Gold, and Justin E. Trivax. "Changes in Renal Markers and Acute Kidney Injury after Marathon Running." *Nephrology* 16, no. 2 (2011): 194–99. www.ncbi.nlm.nih.gov/pubmed/21272132.

McHugh, Kathryn, Bridget A. Hearon, and Michael W. Otto. "Cognitive-behavioral Therapy for Substance Use Disorders." *Psychiatric Clinics of North America* 33, no. 3 (2010): 511–25.

McKenzie, Donald C. "Markers of Excessive Exercise." *Canadian Journal of Applied Physiology* 24, no. 1 (1999): 66–73.

McKenzie, Shelly. *Getting Physical: The Rise of Fitness Culture in America*. Lawrence: University Press of Kansas, 2013.

McLean, Daniel, and Amy Hurd. *Kraus' Recreation and Leisure in Modern Society*. Burlington, MA: Jones & Bartlett Learning, 2012.

McNamara, Justin, and Marita P. McCabe. "Striving for Success or Addiction? Exercise Dependence among Elite Australian Athletes." *Journal of Sports Sciences* 30, no. 8 (2012): 755–66. DOI:10.1080/02640414.2012.667879.

Mechikoff, Robert A., and Stephen Estes. *A History and Philosophy of Sport and Physical Education*. 3rd ed. Boston: McGraw Hill, 2002.

Merglen, Arnaud, Aline Flatz, Richard E Bélanger, Pierre-André Michaud, and Joan-Carles Suris. "Weekly Sport Practice and Adolescent Well-being." *Archives of Disease in Childhood* 99, no. 3 (2013): 208–10. DOI:10.1136/archdischild-2013-303729.

Metlay, Grischa. "Federalizing Medical Campaigns against Alcoholism and Drug Abuse." *Milbank Quarterly* 91, no. 1 (2013): 123–62. DOI:10.1111/milq.12004.

Michaelides, Andreas P., Dimitris Soulis, Charalambos Antoniades, Alexios S. Antonopoulous, Antigoni Miliou, Nikolaos Ioakeimidis, Evangelos I. Chatzistamatiou, Constantinos Bakogiannis, Kyriakoula Marinou, Charalampos I. Liakos, and Christodoulos Stefanadis. "Exercise Duration as a Determinant of Vascular Function and Antioxidant Balance in Patients with Coronary Artery Disease." *Heart* 97, no. 10 (2011): 832–37. DOI:10.1136/hrt.2010.209080.

Mond, Jonathan M., Phillipa J. Hay, Bryan Rodgers, and Cathy Owen. "An Update on the Definition of 'Excessive Exercise' in Eating Disorders Research." *International Journal of Eating Disorders* 39, no. 2 (2006): 147–53. DOI:10.1002/eat.20214.

Mond, Jonathan M., and Rachel M. Calogero. "Excessive Exercise in Eating Disorder Patients and Healthy Women." *Australian and New Zealand Journal of Psychiatry* 43, no. 3 (2009): 227–34. DOI:10.1080/00048670802653323.

Mond, Jonathan M., Tricia C. Myers, Ross Crosby, Phillipa Hay, and James Mitchell. "Excessive Exercise and Eating-disordered Behaviour in Young Adult Women: Further Evidence from a Primary Care Sample." *European Eating Disorders Review* 16, no. 3 (2008): 215–21. DOI:10.1002/erv.855.

Mónok, Kata, Krisztina Berczik, Róbert Urbán, Attila Szabó, Mark D. Griffiths, Judit Farkas, Anna Magi, Andrea Eisinger, Tamás Kurimay, Gyöngyi Kökönyei, Bernadette Kun, Borbála Paksi, and Zsolt Demetrovics. "Psychometric Properties and Concurrent Validity of Two Exercise Addiction Measures: A Population Wide Study." *Psychology of Sport and Exercise* 13, no. 6 (2012): 739–46. DOI:10.1016/j.psychsport.2012.06.003.

Moore, Kevin. "The Six Most Shockingly Irresponsible 'Fitspiration' Photos." REEMBODY. http://reembody.me/2013/09/10/the-6-most-shockingly-irresponsible-fitspiration-photos. Last modified September 10, 2013. Accessed March 25, 2014.

Morgan, W. P. "Negative Addiction in Runners." *Physician and Sportsmedicine* 7, no. 7 (1979): 57–70.

Morgan, William P., Patrick J. O'Connor, Phillip B. Sparling, and Russ R. Pate. "Psychological Characterizations of the Elite Female Distance Runner." *International Journal of Sports Medicine* 8, suppl. no. 2 (1987): 124–31.

National Association of Anorexia Nervosa. "General Information about Eating Disorders." www.anad.org/get-information/about-eating-disorders/general-information. Accessed March 26, 2014.

National Counsel on Alcoholism. "Criteria for the Diagnosis of Alcoholism." *The American Journal of Psychiatry* 129, no. 2 (1972): 127–35.

National Institute on Drug Abuse. The Science of Drug Abuse and Addiction. "DrugFacts: Anabolic Steroids." www.drugabuse.gov/publications/drugfacts/anabolic-steroids. Last modified July 2012. Accessed February 22, 2014.

Nattiv, Aurelia, Anne B. Loucks, Melinda M. Manore, Charlotte F. Sanborn, Jorunn Sundgot-Borgen, and Michelle P. Warren. "American College of Sports Medicine Position Stand: The Female Athlete Triad." *Medicine and Science in Sports and Exercise* 39, no. 10 (2007): 1867–82.

Neff, Kristin. *Self-compassion*. New York: HarperCollins, 2011.

Ng, Louisa W., Daniel P. Ng, and Wai P. Wong. "Is Supervised Exercise Training Safe in Patients with Anorexia Nervosa? A Meta-analysis." *Physiotherapy* 99, no. 1 (2013): 1–11. DOI:10.1016/j.physio.2012.05.006.

O'Keefe, James H., and Carl J. Lavie. "Run for Your Life . . . at a Comfortable Speed and Not Too Far." *Heart* 99, no. 8 (2013): 516–19. DOI:10.1136/heartjnl-2012-302886.

Olivardia, Roberto. "Muscle Dysmorphia: Characteristics, Assessment, and Treatment." In *The Muscular Ideal: Psychological, Social, and Medical Perspectives*, edited by J. Kevin Thompson and Guy Cafri, 123–39. Washington, DC: American Psychological Association, 2007.

Orford, Jim. "Addiction as Excessive Appetite." *Addiction* 96, no. 1 (2001): 15–31. DOI:10.1080/09652140020016932.

Padwa, Howard, and Jacob Cunningham. *Addiction: A Reference Encyclopedia*. Santa Barbara, CA: Greenwood Publishing Group, 2010.

Pelliccia, Antonio, Barry J. Maron, Antonio Spataro, Michael A. Proschan, and Paolo Spirito. "The Upper Limit of Physiologic Cardiac Hypertrophy in Highly Trained Elite Athletes." *The New England Journal of Medicine* 324, no. 5 (1991): 295–301. DOI:10.1056/NEJM199101313240504.

Pelliccia, Antonio, Barry J. Maron, Fernando M. Di Paolo, Alessandro Biffi, Filippo M. Quattrini, Cataldo Pisicchio, Alessangra Roselli, Stefano Caselli, and Franco Culasso. "Prevalence and Clinical Significance of Left Atrial Remodeling in Competitive Athletes." *Journal of the American College of Cardiology* 46, no. 4 (2005): 690–96. DOI:10.1016/j.jacc.2005.04.052.

Peñas-Lledó, Eva, Francisco J. Vaz Leal, and Glen Waller. "Excessive Exercise in Anorexia Nervosa and Bulimia Nervosa: Relation to Eating Characteristics and General Psychopathology." *International Journal of Eating Disorders* 31, no. 4 (2002): 370–75. DOI:10.1002/eat.10042.

Peternelj Tina-Tinkara, and Jeff S. Coombes. "Antioxidant Supplementation during Exercise Training: Beneficial or Detrimental?" *Sports Medicine* 41, no. 12 (2011): 1043–69. DOI:10.2165/11594400-000000000-00000.

Philips, Janine M., and Murray J. N. Drummond. "An Investigation into the Body Image Perception, Body Satisfaction and Exercise Expectations of Male Fitness Leaders: Implications for Professional Practice." *Leisure Studies* 20, no. 2 (2001): 95–105.

Phillips, Murray G., and Alexander Paul Roper. "History of Physical Education." In *Handbook of Physical Education*, edited by David Kirk, Doune Macdonald, Mary O'Sullivan, 123–41. Burlington, MA: Jones & Bartlett Learning, 2015.

Pluim, Babette M., Aeilko H. Zwinderman, Arnoud van der Laarse, and Ernst E. van der Wall. "The Athlete's Heart: A Meta-analysis of Cardiac Structure and Function." *Circulation* 101, no. 3 (2000): 336–44. DOI:10.1161/01.CIR.101.3.336.

Powell, Lisa M., Sandy Slater, and Frank J. Chaloupka. "The Relationship between Community Physical Activity Settings and Race, Ethnicity and Socioeconomic Status." *Evidence-based Prevention Medicine* 1, no. 2 (2004): 135–44.

Prochaska, James O., and Wayne F. Velicer. "The Transtheoretical Model of Health Behavior Change." *American Journal of Health Promotion* 12, no. 1 (1997): 38–48.

Putney, Clifford. *Muscular Christianity: Manhood and Sports in Protestant America, 1880–1920.* Cambridge, MA: Harvard University Press, 2001.

Ravaldi, Claudia, Alfredo Vannacci, Teresa Zucchi, Edoardo Mannucci, Pier Luigi Cabras, Maura Boldrini, Loriana Murciano, Carlo Maria Rotella, and Valdo Ricca. "Eating Disorders and Body Image Disturbances among Ballet Dancers, Gymnasium Users and Body Builders." *Psychopathology* 36, no. 5 (2003): 247–54. DOI:10.1159/000073450.

Reynolds, Gretchen. "Crash and Burnout." *The New York Times.* www.nytimes.com/2008/03/02/sports/playmagazine/02play-physed.html?pagewanted=all. Accessed March 2, 2008.

Richardson, Sean O., Mark B. Andersen, and Tony Morris. *Overtraining Athletes: Personal Journeys in Sport.* Champaign, IL: Human Kinetics, 2008.

Rosenberg, Morris, and Leonard I. Pearlin. "Social Class and Self-esteem among Children and Adults." *American Journal of Sociology* 84, no. 1 (1978): 53–77.

Rosenberg, Nathan. "MMPI Alcoholism Scales." *Journal of Clinical Psychology* 28, no. 4 (1972): 515–22. DOI:10.1002/1097-4679(197210)28:4&#60515::AID-JCLP2270280421&#623.0.CO;2-N.

Roy, Alec. "Childhood Trauma and Neuroticism as an Adult: Possible Implication for the Development of the Common Psychiatric Disorders and Suicidal Behaviour." *Psychological Medicine* 32, no. 8 (2002): 1471–74. DOI:10.1017/S0033291702006566.

Ruiz, Francisco J. "Acceptance and Commitment Therapy versus Traditional Cognitive Behavioral Therapy: A Systematic Review and Meta-analysis of Current Empirical Evidence." *International Journal of Psychology & Psychological Therapy* 12, no. 2 (2012): 333–57.

Russell, Wendy. "Yoga and Vertebral Arteries." *British Medical Journal* 1, no. 5801 (1972): 685.

Samuels, Donald J., and Muriel Samuels. "Low Self-concept as a Cause of Drug Abuse." *Journal of Drug Education* 4, no. 4 (1974): 421–38. DOI:10.2190/VJHU-MRAR-NLG6-1XBH.

Sarramon, Christine, Hélène Verdoux, Laurent Schmitt, and Marc-Louis Bourgeois. "Addiction and Personality Traits: Sensation Seeking, Anhedonia, Impulsivity." *L'Encéphale* 25, no. 6 (1999): 569–75.

Schmied, Christian, and Mats Borjesson. "Sudden Cardiac Death in Athletes." *Journal of Internal Medicine* 275, no. 2 (2014): 93–103. DOI:10.1111/joim.12184.

Schultz, Wolfram. "Reward Signaling by Dopamine Neurons." *The Neuroscientist* 7, no. 4 (2001): 293–302. DOI:10.1177/107385840100700406.

Schwartz, Jonathan G., Stacia Merkel-Kraus, Sue Duval, Kevin Harris, Gretchen Peichel, John R. Lesser, Thomas Knickelbine, Bjorn Flygenring, Terry R. Longe, Catherine Pastorius, William R. Roberts, Stephen C. Oesterle, and Robert S. Schwartz. "Does Elite Athleticism Enhance or Inhibit Coronary Artery Plaque Formation? A Prospective Multidetector CTA Study of Men Completing Marathons for at Least 25 Consecutive Years." Paper presented at the American College of Cardiology 2010 Scientific Sessions, Atlanta, GA (2010): 1271–330. www.abstractsonline.com/Plan/ViewAbstract.aspx?mID=2444&sKey=747bc0a9-d52f-4671-a6c7-e189fbc76e0a&cKey=8d57d453-a124-4c89-a1d0-da559dbfa754&mKey=7a9907ef-0b49-4421-a7ae-7e7f1ebb9402. Accessed March 12, 2014.

Schwarz, Lothar, and Wilfried Kindermann. "Changes in β-Endorphin Levels in Response to Aerobic and Anaerobic Exercise." *Sports Medicine* 13, no. 1 (1992): 25–36. DOI:10.2165/00007256-199213010-00003.

———. "Beta-endorphin, Adrenocorticotropic Hormone, Cortisol and Catecholamines during Aerobic and Anaerobic Exercise." *European Journal of Applied Physiology* 61, nos. 3–4 (1990): 165–71. DOI:10.1007/BF00357593.

Setiawan, Elaine, Robert O. Pihl, Alain Dagher, Hera Schlagintweit, Kevin F. Casey, Chawki Benkelfat, and Marco Leyton. "Differential Striatal Dopamine Responses Following Oral Alcohol in Individuals at Varying Risk for Dependence." *Alcoholism: Clinical and Experimental Research* 38, no. 1 (2014): 126–34. DOI:10.1111/acer.12218.

Shangold, Mona M., and H. S. Levine. "The Effect of Marathon Training upon Menstrual Function." *American Journal of Obstetrics and Gynecology* 143, no. 8 (1982): 862–69.

Shannahoff-Khalsa, David, Laura E. Ray, Saul Levine, Christopher C. Gallen, Barb J. Schwartz, and John J. Sidorowich. "Randomized Controlled Trial of Yogic Meditation Techniques for Patients with Obsessive Compulsive Disorder." *CNS Spectrums* 4, no. 12 (1999): 34–47.

Sharp, Katie. "A Review of Acceptance and Commitment Therapy with Anxiety Disorders." *International Journal of Psychology & Psychological Therapy* 12, no. 3 (2012): 359–72.

Sheppard, Mary N. "The Fittest Person in the Morgue?" *Histopathology* 60, no. 3 (2012): 381–96. DOI:10.1111/j.1365-2559.2011.03852.x.

Siedentop, Daryl. *Introduction to Physical Education, Fitness, and Sport.* 7th ed. New York: McGraw-Hill Higher Education, 2009. http://highered.mcgraw-hill.com/sites/dl/free/0073376515/669664/Siedentop7e_ch02.pdf. Accessed February 24, 2014.

Sinha, Rajita. "Chronic Stress, Drug Use, and Vulnerability to Addiction." *Annals of the New York Academy of Sciences* 1141 (2008): 105–30. DOI:10.1196/annals.1441.030.

Slay, Heather A., Jumi Hayaki, Melissa A. Napolitano, and Kelly D. Brownell. "Motivations for Running and Eating Attitudes in Obligatory versus Nonobligatory Runners." *International Journal of Eating Disorders* 23, no. 3 (1998): 267–75. DOI:10.1002/(SICI)1098-108X(199804)23:3&#60267::AID-EAT4&#623.0.CO;2-H.

Smith, David E. "Editor's Note: The Process Addictions and the New ASAM Definition of Addiction." *Journal of Psychoactive Drugs* 44, no. 1 (2012): 1–4. DOI:10.1080/02791072.2012.662105.

Smith, David K., Bruce D. Hale, and David J. Collins. "Measurement of Exercise Dependence in Bodybuilders," *Journal of Sport Medicine and Physical Fitness* 38, no. 1 (1998): 66–74.

Smolak, Linda, and Sarah K. Murnen. "A Meta-analytic Examination of the Relationship between Child Sexual Abuse and Eating Disorders." *International Journal of Eating Disorders* 31, no. 2 (2002): 136–50. DOI:10.1002/eat.10008.

Smoliga, James M., Joseph A. Baur, and Heather A. Hausenblas. "Resveratrol and Health: A Comprehensive Review of Human Clinical Studies." *Molecular Nutrition and Food Research* 55, no. 8 (2011): 1129–41. DOI:10.1002/mnfr.201100143.

Springer, Kristen W., Jennifer Sheridan, Daphne Kuo, and Molly Carnes. "The Long-term Health Outcomes of Childhood Abuse." *Journal of General Internal Medicine* 18, no. 10 (2003): 864–70. DOI:10.1046/j.1525-1497.2003.20918.x.

Sussman, Steve, Nadra Lisha, and Mark Griffiths. "Prevalence of the Addictions: A Problem of the Majority or the Minority?" *Evaluation & the Health Professions* 34, no. 1 (2011): 3–56. DOI:10.1177/0163278710380124.

Symons Downs, Danielle, Heather A. Hausenblas, and Claudio R. Nigg. "Factorial Validity and Psychometric Examination of the Exercise Dependence Scale—Revised." *Measurement in Physical Education and Exercise Science* 8, no. 4 (2004): 183–201. DOI:10.1207/s15327841mpee0804_1.

Szabó, Attila. "Physical Activity and Psychological Dysfunction." In *Physical Activity and Psychological Well-being*, edited by Stuart J. H. Biddle, Ken Fox, and Steve Boutcher, 130–53. New York: Routledge, 2000.

———. "The Impact of Exercise Deprivation on Well-being of Habitual Exercisers." *Australian Journal of Science and Medicine in Sport* 27, no. 3 (1995): 68–75.

Szabó, Attila, and Mark D. Griffiths. "Exercise Addiction in British Sport Science Students." *International Journal of Mental Health and Addiction* 5, no. 1 (2007): 25–28.

Taranis, Lorin, and Caroline Meyer. "Associations between Specific Components of Compulsive Exercise and Eating-disordered Cognitions and Behaviors among Young Women." *The International Journal of Eating Disorders* 44, no. 5 (2011): 452–58. DOI:10.1002/eat.20838.

Taranis, Lorin, Stephen Touyz, and Caroline Meyer. "Disordered Eating and Exercise: Development and Preliminary Validation of the Compulsive Exercise Test (CET)." *European Eating Disorders Review* 19, no. 3 (2011): 256–68. DOI:10.1002/erv.1108.

Teasdale, John D., Zindel V. Segal, J. Mark G. Williams, Valerie A. Ridgeway, Judith M. Soulsby, and Mark A. Lau. "Prevention of Relapse/Recurrence in Major Depression by Mindfulness-based Cognitive Therapy." *Journal of Consulting and Clinical Psychology* 68, no. 4 (2000): 615–23. DOI:10.1037/0022-006X.68.4.615.

Terret, Thierry, and J. A. Mangan. *Sport, Militarism and the Great War*. New York: Routledge, 2012.

Terry, Annabel, Attila Szabó, and Mark D. Griffiths. "The Exercise Addiction Inventory: A New Brief Screening Tool." *Addiction Research and Theory* 12, no. 5 (2004): 489–99. DOI:10.1080/16066350310001637363.

Thein-Nissenbaum, Jill. "Long Term Consequences of the Female Athlete Triad." *Maturitas* 75, no. 2 (2013): 107–12.

Uebleis, Christopher, Alexander Becker, Ines Griesshammer, Paul Cumming, Christoph Becker, Michael Schmidt, Peter Bartenstein, and Marcus Hacker. "Stable Coronary Artery Disease: Prognostic Value of Myocardial Perfusion SPECT in Relation to Coronary Calcium Scoring—Long-term Follow-up." *Radiology* 252, no. 3 (2009): 682–90. DOI:10.1148/radiol.2531082137.

U.S. Department of Health and Human Services. "Physical Activity Guidelines for Americans." www.health.gov/paguidelines/guidelines/chapter6.aspx. Last modified October 16, 2008. Accessed March 26, 2014.

Vanholder, Raymond, Mehmet Sükrü Sever, Ekrem Erek, and Norbert Lameire. "Rhabdomyolysis." *Journal of the American Society of Nephrology* 11, no. 8 (2000): 1553–61.

Vlachopoulos, Charalambos, Despina Kardara, Aris Anastasakis, Katerina Baou, Dimitrios Terentes-Printzios, Dimitris Tousoulis, and Christodoulos Stefanadis. "Arterial Stiffness and Wave Reflections in Marathon Runners." *American Journal of Hypertension* 23, no. 9 (2010): 974–79. DOI:10.1038/ajh.2010.99.

Wade, George N., and Juli E. Jones. "Neuroendocrinology of Nutritional Infertility." *American Journal of Physiology: Regulatory, Integrative and Comparative Physiology* 287, no. 6 (2004): R1277–96. www.ncbi.nlm.nih.gov/pubmed/15528398.

Wallet, Max. "Deux cas d'anorexie hystérique." In *Nouvelle Iconographie de la Salpêtrière*, edited by. J.-M. Charcot. Paris: 1892.

Weinstein, Aviv, and Yitzhak Weinstein. "Exercise Addiction—Diagnosis, Bio-psychological Mechanisms and Treatment Issues." *Current Pharmaceutical Design* 20 (2014): 1–8. DOI:10.2174/13816128113199990614.

Wexler, Bruce E., Christopher H. Gottschalk, Robert K. Fulbright, Isak Prohovnik, Cheryl M. Lacadie, Bruce J. Rounsaville, and John C. Gore. "Functional Magnetic Resonance Imaging of Cocaine Craving." *The American Journal of Psychiatry* 158, no. 1 (2001): 86–95. DOI:10.1176/appi.ajp.158.1.86.

Wilson, Mathew, Rory O'Hanlon, Satyendra K. Prasad, A. Deighan, Peter D. Macmillan, Dave Oxborough, Richard Godfrey, Gillian Smith, Alicia Maceira, Sanjay Sharma, Keith P. George, and Gregory P. White. "Diverse Patterns of Myocardial Fibrosis in Lifelong, Veteran Endurance Athletes." *Journal of Applied Physiology* 110, no. 6 (2011): 1622–26.

Wolitzky-Taylor, Kate B., Joanna J. Arch, David Rosenfield, and Michelle G. Craske. "Moderators and Non-specific Predictors of Treatment Outcome for Anxiety Disorders: A Comparison of Cognitive Behavioral Therapy to Acceptance and Commitment Therapy." *Journal of Consulting and Clinical Psychology* 80, no. 5 (2012): 786–99. DOI:10.1037/a0029418.

Wood, Joanne V., W. Q. Elaine Perunovic, and John W. Lee. "Positive Self-statements: Power for Some, Peril for Others." *Psychological Science* 20, no. 7 (2009): 860–66. DOI:10.1111/j.1467-9280.2009.02370.x.

Xenophon. *Hellenica*. c. 370 BCE. Quoted in Stephen G. Miller, *Arete: Greek Sports from Ancient Sources*. Berkeley: University of California Press, 1991.

———. *Memorabilia*. c. 371 B.C. Quoted in E. Norman Gardiner, *Athletics in the Ancient World*. London: Oxford University Press, 1930.

Yates, Alayne. *Compulsive Exercise and the Eating Disorders*. New York: Brunner/Mazel, 1991.

Zettle, Robert D. "The Evolution of a Contextual Approach to Therapy: From Comprehensive Distancing to ACT." *International Journal of Behavioral Consultation and Therapy* 1, no. 2 (2005): 77–89.

Zglerska, Aleksandra, David Rabago, Neharika Chawla, Kenneth Kushner, Robert Koehler, and Alan Marlatt. "Mindfulness Meditation for Substance Use Disorders: Systematic Review." *Substance Abuse* 30, no. 4 (2009): 266–94. DOI:10.1080/08897070903250019.

Zhao, Yafu, and William Encinos. "Hospitalizations for Eating Disorders from 1999 to 2006." Statistical Brief #70. *Healthcare Cost and Utilization Project (HCUP)*. Rockville, MD: Agency for Healthcare Research and Quality, January 2011. www.hcup-us.ahrq.gov/reports/statbriefs/sb70.jsp.

Zukin, Sharon, and Jennifer Smith Maguire. "Consumers and Consumption." *Annual Review of Sociology* 30 (2004): 173–97. DOI:10.1146/annurev.soc.30.012703.110553.

INDEX